Diabetes?
No Problema!

Diabetes?
No Problema!

The Latino's Guide
to Living Well
with Diabetes

Sheri R. Colberg, PhD

Leonel Villa-Caballero, MD, PhD

Latino researcher and director of the Latino Initiative of
"Taking Control of Your Diabetes"

With a foreword by
Chef LaLa

Alameda Free Library
1550 Oak Street
Alameda, CA 94501

A Member of the Perseus Books Group

Designed by Brent Wilcox
Set in 11.25 point Adobe Caslon by the Perseus Books Group

Library of Congress Cataloging-in-Publication Data
Colberg, Sheri, 1963-
    Diabetes? No problema! : the Latino's guide to living well with diabetes / Sheri R. Colberg and Leonel Villa-Caballero ; with a foreword by Chef LaLa. — 1st ed.
        p.   cm.
    Includes bibliographical references and index.
    ISBN 978-0-7382-1315-6 (alk. paper)
    1. Diabetes—Popular works.   2. Hispanic Americans—Diseases—Popular works.
I. Villa-Caballero, Leonel.   II. Title.
    RC660.4.C646 2009
    616.4'62--dc22
                                                                                    2009012714

First Da Capo Press edition 2009

Published by Da Capo Press
A Member of the Perseus Books Group
www.dacapopress.com

Da Capo Press books are available at special discounts for bulk purchases in the U.S. by corporations, institutions, and other organizations. For more information, please contact the Special Markets Department at the Perseus Books Group, 2300 Chestnut Street, Suite 200, Philadelphia, PA, 19103, or call (800) 810-4145, ext. 5000, or e-mail special.markets@perseusbooks.com.

10 9 8 7 6 5 4 3 2 1

For my loving and supportive husband, Ray Ochs,
and my three wonderful sons—may you also follow
the advice we give in this book to remain
diabetes-free throughout your lives.
—SC

For Olga Alicia, my dear partner in dreams and life;
for Nonita, wherever you are; and for all those Latino
patients who patiently taught me the value of
compassion and love.
—LVC

CONTENTS

FOREWORD by Chef LaLa   ix

INTRODUCTION Why Latinos Need to Take on
the Diabetes *Problema* Now   xiii

1 *Living* La Vida Buena *with Diabetes in a Latino Culture*   1

2 *Understanding Body Fat, Fitness, and Diabetes*   21

3 *Going Beyond the Latino Diet*   37

4 *Choosing Supplements Wisely*   69

5 *Moving More for Your Body, Heart, and Mind*   101

6 *Learning How to Exercise Safely and Effectively*   121

7 *Treating Your Diabetes Right: Monitoring and Medications*   149

8 *Controlling Stress, Depression, and Your Emotions*   171

9 *Limiting Diabetes-Related Health Problems*   191

10 *Staying on the Road to Good Health*   207

CONCLUSION Taking on Diabetes . . . and Winning 221

APPENDIX A Important Websites for Diabetic
(and Prediabetic) Latinos 223

APPENDIX B Glycemic Index and Glycemic Load of
Common Foods 227

SUGGESTED READING 231

SELECTED REFERENCES BY CHAPTER 233

ACKNOWLEDGMENTS 253

ABOUT THE AUTHORS 255

INDEX 257

FOREWORD

by Chef LaLa
(Laura Diaz-Brown)

Twenty years ago, the title of this book, *Diabetes? No Problema!* would have been an oxymoron. In the past, a diabetes diagnosis was often a cause for hopelessness. Thank goodness that has changed! We've come a long way in our understanding of how a variety of foods—not just sugar—are converted to glucose in the body. And now we know that exercise is critical to diabetes prevention and management. Living with diabetes today is, in fact, no problema.

However, despite what we know about the disease, how to ward it off, and how to prevent complications, the number of new cases is rising along with the death rate. Latinos are at special risk. As authors Sheri R. Colberg and Leonel Villa-Caballero point out, more than 10 percent of all Mexican Americans twenty years or older have diabetes. That's almost double the rate of non-Hispanic whites. Other Latinos have somewhat lower rates, but still higher than non-Hispanic whites.

Although I don't have diabetes myself, it's hard to shake those numbers from my head. I know how devastating it is to watch a loved one struggle to manage the illness and then suffer through the later stages of the disease. I lost both of my grandmothers and one of my grandfathers to complications of diabetes. Seven of my father's eight brothers are currently living with diabetes. My dad has it too.

Though this book is geared toward Latinos, the advice it contains is applicable to anyone, especially those with strong cultural ties. In my work as a chef and certified nutritionist, I hear all the time from people belonging to a variety of ethnic groups that they want to eat healthier without giving up the comfort and flavor of their traditional cuisine. Latinos will say, "Well, my grandmother always made that with lard. That's how it's been done for generations." While it's true that our parents and grandparents cooked for us with the intention of giving us the best, do you think they would have used certain ingredients, like lard, if they had known the long-term consequences of doing so?

It's okay to tweak traditional recipes. It's okay to make healthier choices without sacrificing the rich culture that we hold dear. After all, we are the next generation of *abuelos* and *abuelitas*. We have the power to create new traditions from old—so we can stop being a statistic. Our *abuelos* came to this country because they wanted for us to have a better life. A better life for me, frankly, is having my dad around for a good long time. And I personally want to be around a good long time for my son and his children.

If you have diabetes or if you're reading this because you know someone who has it, what better time to build a healthier lifestyle that involves the entire *familia*? There's no need to feel guilty because you have certain dietary needs. Eating well to manage or prevent disease is not the same as going on a diet. In fact, I loathe the word "diet" because it implies deprivation. There are many foods that you can eat without sacrificing *sabor*. Just switching to different cooking methods, such as broiling, steaming, or baking, or eating less meat—which were the norm in many of our cultures before modern-day influences were introduced—can have a tremendous impact on health. And think about the native produce of Mexico, Central and South America, and the Caribbean that's now available on our store shelves: *maracuyá, tamarindo, jocote.* Something that comes in its own package, the way nature intended, is always an excellent choice.

You also have the opportunity to create new family traditions involving exercise, which is critical for your long-term well-being. Going for a walk after dinner is a great time to catch up on the day's events. Bicycling with your children can be fun and relaxing. If you really want to honor our heritage, put on some music and dance. There's no reason you can't exercise *con sazón.* But please, don't make the excuse that you don't have time. Because if you don't have time to take care of yourself now, then be prepared to make a lot of time for disease later. Being sick, having a heart attack, going to the hospital—all of that takes time. *Mejor prevenir que lamentar.*

Latinos especially have difficulty admitting their condition, discussing it with others, and getting help. So, if you haven't already, surround yourself with a team of medical professionals who make you feel comfortable. Then make the lifestyle changes necessary to manage your blood sugar. When you face diabetes head-on and take control of the daily decisions that affect your health, the people around you will know how to support you. The beauty of our culture is the importance we place on *familia.* We go through this together.

For those of you who are reading this book, I applaud you. Even if you don't have diabetes yourself, or even if you belong to a different ethnic group, you'll find these pages brimming with useful information. The important thing is to take hold of your condition. You need to ask yourself, Do I have diabetes or does diabetes have me? You can have diabetes and still have it all!

INTRODUCTION

Why Latinos Need to Take on the Diabetes Problema *Now*

The latest findings about who has and who will get diabetes are alarming. At last estimate in 2007, almost 24 million people in the United States already had diabetes, and a quarter of them had no idea that they did. A conservative estimate of the number of diabetic Americans by the year 2030 is over 30 million, but it's likely to turn out to be much higher than that. Currently over two and a half million Latinos (about 10 percent of the people afflicted with diabetes in the U.S.) are believed to have diabetes as well. A child born in the new millennium is estimated to have a one in three chance of developing diabetes at some point; for certain ethnic minorities, the risk is closer to one in two. Unfortunately Hispanics fall into the second risk category.

How do you know if you're considered Latino, Hispanic, or both?

How do you know if your ethnic group is Latino, Hispanic, or both? By definition, ethnic groups are classified according to common racial, national, tribal, religious, linguistic, or cultural origin or background. According to that definition, Hispanics are people of Latin American descent living in the United States, particularly those with origins in Mexico, Puerto Rico, Cuba, or other Central or South American countries. Latinos are individuals of Latin American descent whose ancestors came from any of the countries south of the United States. Confused about the difference? So are we. Apparently the term "Hispanic" was created by the U.S. federal government in the early 1970s in an attempt to provide a common denominator to a large but diverse population with connections to the Spanish language and a culture from a Spanish-speaking country. "Latino" is becoming more accepted within this minority group itself, but in this book we will use the two terms interchangeably to cover everyone.

Latinos of any race now comprise America's largest minority group (slightly edging out African Americans) and remain the fastest-growing segment of the population. As of the 2000 census, more than 44 million Latinos were living in the United States, accounting for almost 15 percent of the total population, and they are expected to comprise 30 percent of Americans by the middle of this century. A diverse and heterogeneous group, we Latinos share a common ancestry, language, and culture, even with a mix of European, African, Asian, and Native American blood.

Your risk for developing diabetes is higher than average

Unfortunately all Latinos share an increased incidence of diabetes regardless of ethnic mix. We Latinos are second only to Native Americans in having the highest incidence of diabetes in the United States, and we get it at earlier ages than other populations. Among Puerto Ricans and Mexican Americans, the age of onset is thirty to fifty years. More than 10 percent of all Mexican Americans twenty or older have diabetes, which is almost twice the rate of non-Hispanic whites of a similar age. Cuban Americans have a slightly lower rate of diabetes than Mexican Americans and Puerto Ricans, but still higher than non-Hispanic whites. Thus health concerns like diabetes in Latino communities can have serious and wide-reaching implications for the national health care system and America's collective health, not to mention the health of any of your relatives living south of the United States in your family's native country.

Why is your diabetes risk higher if you're Latino? It may have to do with the genes you inherited, but obviously there are other factors (e.g., lifestyle choices) that may be equally, if not more, important in the disease's development. Fortunately, we now know that type 2 diabetes is largely preventable even if you have a higher risk due to your ethnicity, as demonstrated by a study of over 3,200 people concluded in 2003. All of the individuals participating in the Diabetes Prevention Program had prediabetes and were at high risk of developing the disease. At least 15 percent were Latinos, and the results showed that lifestyle choices—diet, exercise, and body weight—can make it possible to delay or prevent diabetes onset in two out of every three Hispanic individuals, more than when all ethnic groups were included. From this study alone you can conclude that while being Latino may increase your risk of getting diabetes, the lifestyle choices that you make likely will have a greater effect.

What can happen if you don't control your diabetes?

Although it's not fun to think about, we think you should be aware of the harm that diabetes can do. Ignoring your diabetes care and claiming ignorance about its possible consequences is not the way to go with this disease. Why? Because diabetes worldwide causes more than 3.2 million deaths per year, or six deaths every minute, and probably more. The leading cause of death in all Americans is heart disease, whether or not you have diabetes. As Latinos, however, we have a higher risk of developing and dying from diabetes, and we're also twice as likely as other populations to experience complications such as heart disease, high blood pressure, blindness, kidney disease, amputations, and nerve damage. This insidious disease is the sixth leading cause of death in Latino communities and the fourth leading cause of death among Latino women and seniors.

Having an elevated blood glucose or blood sugar level can have a tremendously negative impact on your long-term health and enjoyment of life. Diabetes has the potential to rob you, on average, of more than twelve years of your life while reducing the quality of life for twenty or more years.

Diabetes causes other health problems that can severely limit your quality of life. For instance, elevated blood sugar levels over time can damage your eyes, kidneys, and nerves. Poorly controlled diabetes is the leading cause of new cases of blindness among adults, with proliferative diabetic retinopathy (a severe form of diabetic eye disease) alone causing tens of thousands of these new cases in addition to those caused by glaucoma, cataracts, and neuropathy of the optic or eye muscle nerves. Poorly managed diabetes is also the leading cause of kidney disease treated by dialysis and ultimately kidney transplants. Nerve damage can cause numbness in feet or hands, gastroparesis (slowing of the digestion of food), carpal tunnel syndrome, and severe dizziness when standing up, and can lead to toe, foot, and leg amputations. If you're pregnant and have diabetes, your baby can get too big and have a higher risk of birth defects unless you effectively control your blood sugar.

But despite these sobering facts, we're here to reassure you that you can live a long and healthy life with diabetes or prediabetes. The rest of this book will teach you everything you need to know to improve your health through means within your control, like your diet, physical activity, and stress management. The good news is that it's possible for you to start gaining health benefits today. Taking control of your diabetes is important for you and your whole family!

CHAPTER 1

Living La Vida Buena
with Diabetes in
a Latino Culture

If you are reading this book, then you obviously are interested in learning more about how to change *¡Qué problema!* into *¡No problema!* when it comes to diabetes and your health. You've taken the first step toward reducing your risk of getting diabetes and experiencing its potential health problems by making the decision to read this book and learn how to manage your diabetes. Fighting this insidious disease depends on developing greater diabetes-related awareness and spreading education from person to person, community to community. Doing it Latino style is likely going to involve a collective change in the Hispanic community's response to diabetes care and education. Without intervention and a concerted effort, all the diabetes-related management tools in the world aren't going to keep diabetes from negatively affecting

1

the lives of many Latinos—possibly even you or someone in your family.

The different faces of diabetes

Do you know what type of diabetes you or someone you know has? Not everyone develops the same type, but one is definitely more common than all the others. More than 90 percent of people are developing type 2 diabetes, which is largely due to lifestyle habits that promote insulin resistance and other bodily changes that lead to high blood sugar levels. This condition usually results from an inability of the hormone insulin to effectively use blood sugar and then the loss of beta cells that make insulin in your pancreas.

Some of the symptoms of hyperglycemia, or elevated blood sugar levels, include increased thirst, excessive urination, unusual fatigue, blurred vision, unexplained hunger, rapid weight loss, and slow-healing cuts and infections. If you or a loved one have complained recently about excessive thirst, frequent urination, or excessive hunger, you should ask for an appointment with your physician or health care professional to check for diabetes. Often diabetes has more subtle symptoms and may go undetected for some time. Make sure to have your fasting blood sugar levels tested annually.

While many may consider type 2 diabetes a less severe condition than type 1, it is more complex in its origin. For it to develop, you have to have an underlying genetic susceptibility that, when exposed to a variety of social, behavioral, and/or environmental factors, unleashes a latent tendency for diabetes. Some scientific evidence suggests a greater genetic susceptibility for type 2 diabetes among Latinos, apparently due to their mixture of Indian, African, and Caucasian heritages. While this genetic background is undeniably important, the unprecedented increase in cases of people with type 2 diabetes suggests that a bigger cause is a combination of factors that increase insulin resistance—which occurs when your body becomes resistant to the action of the hormone insulin that normally keeps your blood sugars in a normal range, such as a sedentary lifestyle and a poor diet. If you develop type 2 diabetes, you likely have impaired insulin action combined with insulin secretion that is maximal but insufficient. In other words, your body can't make enough insulin to fully overcome your body's resistance to it. Most adults with type 2 diabetes are suffering from some degree of beta cell "burnout," which has led to a diminishing release of insulin over time and rising blood sugar levels. In other words, the beta cells in the pancreas that are responsible for making insulin eventually lose some or all of their ability to do so when exposed to high levels of sugar in your blood over time.

Another 5 to 10 percent have type 1 diabetes, which results from an abnormal immune system response. In this type, specific immune cells (T cells) attack the pancreatic beta cells and destroy them, leaving you unable to produce insulin. This autoimmune process (immune cells killing off parts of your own body) occurs only if you have a genetic predisposition to having it set off by an environmental trigger (e.g., a virus), which causes the body's immune cells (T cells) to destroy the insulin-producing beta cells in the pancreas. Symptoms first appear when about 10 percent of beta cell function remains. Classically, type 1 diabetes is what affects children, except in rare instances. But nowadays more youth are developing type 2, making it difficult to correctly determine the type of diabetes at diagnosis since some of the initial symptoms are similar. To add to the confusion, about half of the cases of type 1 diabetes are now being diagnosed in adults as a slow-onset form called LADA (latent autoimmune diabetes of the adult), or type 1.5.

Since puberty is accompanied by vast elevations in hormones that make insulin resistance worse, type 2 diabetes in youth most often occurs in mid-puberty. Type 1 diabetes also may have its onset during puberty, as rising hormone levels can overtax the ability of any remaining beta cells to produce enough insulin. The similar age at onset can confound an immediate diagnosis of type 2 versus type 1 in youth. Having excess body fat used to be an almost guaranteed indicator of type 2 diabetes, but that is no longer the case as people who develop type 1 are often overweight and can develop an insulin-resistant state resulting from lifestyle choices.

Although you may recognize the classic symptoms of diabetes, they don't necessarily tell you which type of diabetes you have. Additional markers that may assist in diagnosis and determination of diabetes type are present in your blood, including beta cell and insulin autoantibodies, which signal the autoimmunity of type 1, while normal or elevated fasting insulin or C-peptide levels indicative of insulin production point to type 2.

Many women develop gestational diabetes during later pregnancy. This type of diabetes usually disappears after the baby is born, but it signals that your risk for developing type 2 diabetes later in life is greatly elevated. If you have ever given birth to a baby weighing nine pounds or more, then you likely had gestational diabetes during your pregnancy. All pregnant women should be screened for this condition with an oral glucose test no later than twenty-four to twenty-eight weeks into their pregnancy, and possibly even earlier if it has occurred during previous pregnancies.

How diabetes and prediabetes are diagnosed

At present, there are two clinical methods for diagnosing prediabetes and diabetes (see reference values in Table 1.1). The first is measuring

Characteristics of Type 1 Diabetes

- Usually not obese (but can be)
- Often recent (sometimes dramatic) weight loss
- Short duration of symptoms (such as excessive thirst and frequent urination)
- Presence of ketones (in blood or urine) at diagnosis, with about 35 percent with diabetic ketoacidosis (DKA) resulting from excessive ketones
- Often a "honeymoon" period follows initiation of insulin during which insulin needs diminish significantly (or disappear altogether) for a while
- Eventual destruction of the insulin-producing cells, leading to complete dependence on insulin injections
- Ongoing risk of developing diabetic ketoacidosis
- Limited or no family history of type 1 diabetes (but does exist in less than 5 percent of first- or second-degree relatives of diagnosed child)

Characteristics of Type 2 Diabetes

- Overweight at diagnosis (obesity is the hallmark of type 2, but not conclusively)
- Little or no recent weight loss
- Sugar usually in the urine
- Some ketones in the urine at diagnosis in up to 30 percent of cases
- Only 5 percent chance of ketoacidosis at diagnosis
- Little or no excessive thirst and no increased urination
- Strong family history of type 2 diabetes, possibly spanning generations
- At least one parent has diabetes in 45 to 80 percent of cases
- A first- or second-degree relative has diabetes in 74 to 100 percent of cases
- Typically of Hispanic, African American, Asian, Native American, or Pacific Islander descent
- About 90 percent of people with type 2 have dark shiny patches on the skin (acanthosis nigricans), most often found between the fingers or toes, on the back of the neck ("dirty neck"), and in underarm creases
- Polycystic ovary syndrome (PCOS) present in females

your blood sugar levels following an overnight fast (at least eight hours without eating). Normal fasting blood glucose is in the range of 70 to 99 mg/dl, which is simply a measure of the amount of this sugar in a set amount of blood (100 milliliters, or 1 deciliter). For anyone outside of the United States, you'll see your blood sugar values given in millimoles per liter (mmol/L), and a normal value in those units is 3.9 to 5.5 mmol/L. Being on the lower end of the range (near 70 mg/dl or 3.9 mmol/L) first thing in the morning is always better. Prediabetes is diagnosed when your fasting glucose levels are 100 to 125 mg/dl (5.6 to 6.9 mmol/L); this is called impaired fasting glucose (IFG). Diabetes—type 1, 2, or gestational—is having a blood sugar level of 126 mg/dl (7 mmol/L) or above. Alternately, an oral glucose tolerance test (OGTT) involves measuring your blood sugar levels for two to three hours after drinking 75 grams of glucose. This tests your body's ability to respond effectively to a large influx of sugar; elevated sugars are called impaired glucose tolerance (IGT). Depending on how high your blood sugar goes, this test can be used to diagnose diabetes or prediabetes.

In 2009, the American Diabetes Association will be coming out with guidelines to use a third method to diagnose diabetes: the glycated hemoglobin, or hemoglobin A1c test (HbA1c, or A1c for short). The A1c is an indicator of average blood glucose levels over the past two or three months measured by the percent of hemoglobin molecules in the red blood cells with glucose attached. The higher your blood glucose has been, the more glucose will be "stuck" to the hemoglobin. This simple blood test will also diagnose prediabetes and tell you your risk for diabetes, rather than waiting until your fasting blood sugars reach 126 mg/dL to officially diagnose it. Finding out your risk early is important because diabetic complications can occur when your A1c test is at the high end of the normal range.

Table 1.1: Diagnosis of Diabetes or Prediabetes

	Normal	Prediabetes	Diabetes
Fasting Blood Glucose Level, mg/dl (mmol/L)	70–99 (3.9–5.5)	100–125 (5.6–6.9) (IFG, or impaired fasting glucose)	126 (7.0) or higher, on two or more occasions
Oral Glucose Tolerance, mg/dl (mmol/L)	< 140 (7.8) after two hours	140–200 (7.8–11.1) after two hours (IGT, or impaired glucose tolerance)	> 200 (11.1) or higher, on two or more occasions

If you don't have diabetes, can you tell if you have a greater risk of developing it? One of the main symptoms is insulin resistance, and if you are insulin resistant, you can take the steps to reverse it and prevent diabetes. Carrying excess body fat, being physically inactive, and consuming a poor diet suggest that you may be experiencing some degree of reduced insulin action, meaning that your insulin is not working as effectively to keep your blood sugars in check, and it may take more insulin to get the job done.

Two types of body tissue are very sensitive to the effects of insulin: adipose (fat) and muscle. Obesity is associated with an accumulation of fat inside adipose and muscle cells. Muscle is an important storage site for excess glucose and carbohydrates. But when your muscles fill up with excess fat, they become less sensitive to insulin, and your pancreas has to release more insulin to have the same effect. When your level of insulin resistance finally exceeds your ability to secrete enough insulin, you have diabetes. Particularly if you are not physically active, this progression can easily occur over time. However, diabetes is not inevitable even if you already have prediabetes. Exercise increases your muscles' ability to use fat effectively and store extra blood glucose as muscle glycogen, both of which improve insulin action (how effectively insulin stimulates the uptake of blood glucose into those cells). Being active also helps reverse insulin resistance in your liver and reduces the amount of metabolically bad fat stored in your abdomen, which similarly enhances insulin action. (Read more on this topic in Chapter 2.)

In addition to the estimated 24 million cases of diabetes in the United States already, many people have prediabetes. The problem is serious, with an estimated 57 million Americans currently on the brink of developing diabetes if they don't improve their lifestyle—by making dietary improvements and engaging in regular exercise, for starters—in the near future. About 40 percent of adults between forty and seventy-four who were screened in 2000 were diagnosed with prediabetes for having IFG, IGT, or both. About twice as many had IFG (34 percent) than IGT (15 percent), although many of them had both markers of prediabetes.

How you can live la vida buena *with diabetes*

If you have been diagnosed with diabetes, you may be wondering if it is possible for you to live "the good life" (*la vida buena*) despite your diagnosis. The short answer to this question is *sí*. Yes, you can! No matter what type of diabetes you have been diagnosed with—or even if you just want to prevent it—the keys to controlling it, living well, and preventing type 2 diabetes or diabetes-related health complications are within your reach. Effectively controlling any type of diabetes entails daily tasks and choices. But this has become vastly easier in the last few decades with the wide availability of information, new management tools (even online ones), and cutting-edge diabetic medications and technologies. As a result, millions of people now have access to everything they need to manage their diabetes and prediabetes successfully, *if they choose to.*

Latinos face special barriers when it comes to diabetes. Cultural preferences involving food (the types, amounts eaten, and significance of meals) are just one of the ways that Latinos stand out from other minorities. Some would say that specific foods and meal-oriented customs are an integral part of the Latino community, where not eating dessert may be taken as an insult, and everyone expects you to eat cake with your afternoon cup of coffee regardless of how bad it may be for your blood sugar.

Does having diabetes mean that you have to offend others or violate social norms when you forgo that flan at bedtime? If you choose not to involve your family, friends, and acquaintances in your diabetes care, then it may. But in this book we will offer you better ways to handle such situations when you have diabetes or even prediabetes. Regardless of what your favorite forbidden Latino or other food is, you also have the power to change the course of your life and your experiences with diabetes by making small changes like eliminating (or at least reducing) your intake of foods that don't go well with blood sugar control. You can regulate your blood glucose levels to prevent health complications, and in the rest of this book, you'll learn exactly how to do so and read stories about other Latinos who have been successful with managing their diabetes and are truly living *la vida buena*.

GLORIA RODRIGUEZ
A Latina role model for diabetes management

We'd like to introduce you to one shining example of a Latina who has taken diabetes head-on and is winning the war to stay healthy. Her name is Gloria Rodriguez, and she came to the United States from Puerto Rico just to go to college. She stayed, though, and founded Comunicad, Inc., an established public relations and marketing firm based in Washington, D.C.

Gloria has a history of type 2 diabetes in her family, but only as "senior onset." For instance, her uncle was diagnosed at sixty-eight years of age and her mother at seventy-six. When Gloria received the same diagnosis in January 2007 at the age of fifty-five, her first thought was that she was too young to get diabetes. "How can this be happening to me?" she remembers thinking. "I'm not old enough." She had few of the common lifestyle issues that frequently contribute to its onset. She had always watched her diet and had been a vegetarian for many years. "I don't eat french fries, and I have never been a dessert person. I've been good, so why would this happen?" she laments. She used to dance a lot too, doing ballet and modern dance for hours on end when she was younger.

The main contributing factor in Gloria's diabetes may have been her mental stress level. Her experience shows that the effects of stress can be integral in the onset of diabetes. It was only when she was emotionally stressed that she began to feel "funny," which turns out to have corresponded to when her blood sugar levels were elevated. Her stress is understandable. Running a company is stressful, and she travels a lot. Her mother was also sick much of the year before Gloria was diagnosed, causing Gloria to travel to Puerto Rico for extended stays to help care for her. All in all, the stress was too much for her body to handle, and it likely resulted in her diabetes onset, along with having a more sedentary lifestyle at that time than she had ever had in her younger years.

"I had been scheduled to have some surgery earlier this year," Gloria recalls when discussing how her diabetes was found in 2007. "During the preoperative checkups, my blood sugar had been tested, and I was fine. During the routine operation on my gallbladder, there were some problems, and when I awoke from it, I was thirsty." Apparently her blood glucose levels had gone up to 780 mg/dl (although normal levels are less than 100), undoubtedly in part due to the physical stress of surgery. When a doctor came in afterward and asked if she knew that she had diabetes, she responded with denial and disbelief. "I have what?" she remembers saying. "Then you must have given it to me during the operation!"

Having a chronic disease like diabetes is hard for most Latinos to admit; the community as a whole keeps such things hush-hush. Gloria says that admitting to herself that she really has diabetes was one of the hardest things to do. Even her uncle denied his diabetes after his diagnosis until a health problem related to diabetes (a near limb amputation) forced him to accept it and treat it more effectively. As she says, "I usually don't go around with a sign on me announcing that I have diabetes, but if someone asks me, I admit it." She also admits that she's not a run-of-the mill Latina in that respect.

Dealing with food is probably the most difficult part of having diabetes for most Hispanic individuals. Although not much of a dessert eater herself, Gloria understands how important desserts and other foods best avoided by people with diabetes are in the Latino community. As she says, "You can't have two bowls of flan before you go to sleep when you have diabetes, and there is white flour in every meal." Gloria's company has launched several advertising campaigns for manufacturers of diabetes medications like Glucophage (more on this topic in Chapter 7), and she still says that determining how to convince a Latino with diabetes to give up eating certain foods is a challenge. During a campaign to do just that, her company helped launch a TV show that ran for thirteen weeks targeting Latinos. Another featured a TV family where a Latino father developed diabetes and family members got involved in his care by changing their eating patterns, watching the quantity of food eaten, and becoming healthier as a group.

Gloria's development of diabetes and subsequent handling of it exemplifies the issues facing Latinos with regard to diabetes and how to take it on effectively. Soon after her diagnosis, she accepted that she had diabetes and worked to get it under control. One of her strategies was to check her blood sugar levels frequently, often before and after meals (and sometimes every thirty minutes) to get a handle on which foods and situations her body could handle, and which ones it couldn't. She started taking insulin injections with every meal, but soon found that she didn't need that much insulin (she has actually been doing so well that her doctor recently took her off of it). Ironically, she also takes Glucophage, the same medication that she helped promote to Hispanic communities in the United States through her company in recent years. She is truly committed to living well with diabetes, which she intends to do by visiting a nutritionist to learn more about foods and by getting back into exercising regularly, relying on the expertise of a personal trainer for several months to get her started and motivated.

If diabetes has affected you or someone in your family, there is no reason why you can't handle it as effectively as Gloria Rodriguez has. In this book you will read about many more Latinos with diabetes, along with their personal tips and other information essential to helping you live a longer and healthier life despite having diabetes.

The importance of family in the Hispanic culture

You likely know from experience that the traditional Hispanic family is a close-knit group and is often the most important social unit for each family member. Your family likely extends to include aunts, uncles, cousins, grandparents, and even more distant relatives. In most Latino families, the father is the head of the family and the mother is responsible for the home. Everyone sticks together when it comes to helping other members of the family experiencing financial problems, unemployment, health conditions, and other life issues.

These strong family ties extend to traveling as well. For example, someone who travels to another town or city to study or visit can expect to be welcomed into homes of relatives or friends. Family gatherings center on holidays, birthdays, baptisms, first communions, graduations, and weddings, and often they have religious overtones. In the Hispanic world, religion has traditionally played a significant role in daily activity. More than 90 percent of Hispanics are Roman Catholic, although recently other faiths have grown among American Latinos. The church plays a strong role in family life and community affairs and gives spiritual meaning to the culture. For example, local communities often celebrate their unique patron saint's day with greater ceremony than is given to personal birthdays.

Moreover, for many Hispanic families, instilling in their children the importance of honor, good manners, and respect for authority and elders is very important. In most homes, Spanish remains the first language, even if family members are also fluent in English. Why bother to elaborate on these rituals and traditions? These cultural factors can be good or bad when it comes to diabetes management. The more we understand them, the easier it becomes to take on diabetes problems in general and those that pertain to Latinos in particular.

The problem with No hablo inglés *when it comes to effective diabetes care*

A good example of how cultural differences can influence diabetes care is the language barrier. Not understanding the English language can be a huge impediment to patients' obtaining and benefiting from appropriate health care. And even for those who speak a little English (but have no interpreter available at their doctor's office), misdiagnoses and inappropriate medical treatment can result. Even if the doctor understands the problem, you may not be able to understand the medical jargon, treatments, or recommendations. This situation is particularly serious for Latino elderly. About 90 percent speak Spanish in their homes, 56 percent are functionally illiterate in English, and almost 25 percent do not speak English at all.

The real problem is that there aren't enough Spanish-speaking health care professionals around to help Latinos who are not entirely comfortable with the English language. As a result, a great number of the Hispanic elderly never seek out health care or social services because they can't speak or understand English and aren't given literature in their native language. Other studies have shown that Latinos who speak only Spanish have higher levels of A1c, which is indicative of overall higher glucose levels (reflecting poorer blood sugar control), and check their blood glucose levels less often than English-speaking Latinos. In such cases, younger, English-speaking Latinos need to supply translation assistance to recent immigrants to the United States and all who are not yet fully comfortable with English.

Other Latino barriers to good diabetes care

Even if you're fully literate in English, your income and your education level may affect how well you care for your diabetes. Compared with the national average, Latinos have lower income and education levels. Studies have shown that Mexican Americans with a low socioeconomic status have a higher prevalence of obesity and a less favorable distribution of body fat, both of which may contribute to the onset of diabetes. Not having enough money to live well also has serious consequences. If you must focus on daily survival, you may consider health care a lower priority, particularly because of its high cost. When you have health problems with few or no symptoms at first, as is often the case with diabetes and complications like diabetic retinopathy, you may not seek out health care until the problem is advanced and harder to treat or reverse.

For many Latinos, the cost of preventive and frequent checkups, such as an exam to screen for eye problems, is prohibitive because they have to pay for it out of pocket. One study revealed that more than 30 percent of Mexican Americans, 20 percent of Puerto Ricans, and 25 percent of Cuban Americans are uninsured for medical expenses, compared to 20 percent of black Americans and just 10 percent of whites. We don't have to tell you that if you don't have insurance, you're less likely to seek out regular and preventive health care or even visit a doctor annually for a routine physical. We can tell you, though, that your long-term health is likely to suffer without regular checkups, especially if you have diabetes or prediabetes.

The negative impact of certain myths and beliefs among Latinos

There are some popular misconceptions among Latinos related to the causes, treatments, and complications of diabetes. It is very common to hear from your friends or neighbors that diabetes appeared as a consequence of a frightening experience or because someone ate too much candy or sugar. They're not completely right, but they are not entirely wrong either. As we have explained, diabetes occurs as the result of a physiological change in the production of insulin and the way glucose is used in the body. But how well insulin works can be impacted by stress or a poor diet.

Another potential barrier to good heath is that along with religious beliefs, many older Latinos retain cultural biases that focus on fatalism, acceptance, and destiny in dealing with illness. They choose to believe that diabetes is hereditary and determined by God, a disease that must be accepted and endured as punishment for personal sins or those of family members. If you or a family member hold these outdated beliefs, you may be reluctant to seek out health care for diabetic complications, even when routine eye exams may be able to prevent blindness and lower leg amputations. Moreover, Latinos usually express caution about trusting others (e.g., health care professionals) and the help they offer, especially when language barriers exist. We're here to try to convince you that diabetes is not your fault, nor is it a punishment that you or anyone else deserves. We wrote this book to give you the information you need to help you change your thinking, care for yourself more effectively, and seek medical assistance for preventable health problems before they lower your quality of life or shorten it.

Why you need a good doctor or diabetes educator (and where to look)

When it comes to weight loss, diabetes management, or health care in general, you may find group education more useful than individual counseling. Look around for diabetes education classes in your area or even on the Internet. You still need to have a viable relationship with your diabetes doctor, though, for optimal care. For many Latinos, a personal touch in the doctor–patient relationship is crucial to establishing trust. You may need to feel that you can share with your doctors and that they care and listen before you trust them, but such feelings won't arise if you perceive your doctors as impersonal and distant. Some doctors may inadvertently make you feel discriminated against or unwanted, thereby violating your cultural values. A strong sense of pride among the Latino elderly may also affect their ability to accept government assistance in paying for health care because they perceive a welfare stigma attached to it.

Believe us when we tell you that there are doctors who will care for you and your diabetes with respect, dignity, and a personal touch; you may just have to try out more than one to find the perfect doctor for you. If you want to do well with your diabetes, finding a really good doctor or diabetes health care team is critical. How can you tell if you have found good ones? Minimally, they should be up-to-date on the latest research, technologies, medications, and more. If you feel uncomfortable with your doctor's judgment or recommendations, never hesitate to seek out a second opinion about your diabetes care, and switch doctors if you need to in order to find someone who is more knowledgeable or personable.

If doctors who specialize in diabetes (diabetologists or endocrinologists) are not available to you, seek out a good diabetes educator. Nowadays many of them can help you remotely via email, phone, or the Internet. Many diabetes educators are living with diabetes themselves, which serves to increase their awareness of the possible problems you can encounter and how to overcome them. If you don't have access to a computer or the Internet at your home or through someone in your family, try the local library to gain free access to online diabetes education resources (some of which are listed in this chapter; more are given in Appendix A), or even a pay-for-service Internet café.

You can locate diabetes educators on websites like the American Association of Diabetes Educators (www.aadenet.org), which has a diabetes educator locator by city and state, or you can call toll free at (800) 338-3633 for an educator in your area. An example of a long-distance diabetes education group is Integrated Diabetes Services, which is located in Wynnewood, Pennsylvania. It has a team of educators, including certified diabetes educators (CDEs), dietitians, exercise physiologists, and more who can provide personal diabetes coaching and counseling from afar via the Internet (www.integratedservices.com) and telephone (877-SELF-MGT). Insulite Labs (www.insulitelabs.com), Fit4D (www.fit4d.com), and others offer coaching and other diabetes management services.

Even if you can't locate or afford good diabetes care, you can find an abundance of diabetes-related articles and information online, most of it from reputable sources (including www.shericolberg .com). Dr. Leo has recorded some informational videos in Spanish that are available online via the Taking Control of Your Diabetes

Finding More Diabetes and Health Information, Online and in Print

Diabetes magazines and other print materials
- Diabetes Forecast (American Diabetes Association)
- Diabetes Health
- Diabetes Self-Management
- Diabetic Cooking
- Diabetic Gourmet
- Diabetic Living (Better Homes and Gardens)
- Voice of the Diabetic (National Federation of the Blind)

Web resources
- American Diabetes Association: www.diabetes.org (and www.diabetes.org/espanol)
- CDC Division of Diabetes Translation: www.cdc.gov/diabetes
- Children with Diabetes: www.childrenwithdiabetes.com
- David Mendosa, a science writer: www.mendosa.com
- Diabetes Exercise and Sports Association (DESA): www.diabetes-exercise.org
- Diabetes Health online: www.diabeteshealth.com
- Diabetes in Control: www.diabetesincontrol.com
- Diabetes Monitor: www.diabetesmonitor.com
- Diabetes Self-Management online: www.diabetesselfmanagement.com
- Diabetic Cooking online: www.diabeticcooking.com
- dLife—For Your Diabetes Life: www.dlife.com
- Dr. Sheri Colberg's website: www.shericolberg.com
- Hispanopolis: www.hispanopolis.com (a Spanish website with videos on diabetes and more by Dr. Leo)
- Insulite Laboratories: www.insulitelabs.com (diabetes, prediabetes, and weight management)
- Latinos in Shape: www.latinosinshape.com (health and nutrition articles in Spanish)
- Latino Nutrition Coalition: www.latinonutrition.org
- Lifelong Exercise Institute: www.lifelongexercise.com
- National Diabetes Education Program: www.ndep.nih.gov
- National Diabetes Information Clearinghouse: www.diabetes.niddk.nih.gov
- Taking Control of Your Diabetes (TCOYD): www.tcoyd.org (en Español)
- The Diabetes Mall: www.diabetesnet.com (diabetes supplies, books, and information)

Note: Additional web resources are listed in Appendix A.

(www.tcoyd.org) Latino Initiative and on Hispanopolis.com. Watch out for anyone selling products that will easily "cure" your diabetes, though, as these are hucksters trying to make money off of you, and in the end you'll still have diabetes . . . but less cash.

CHAPTER 1: *En pocas palabras* (In a few words)

Latinos of almost all nationalities have an increased risk of developing type 2 diabetes. It is still possible to live *la vida buena* with diabetes, though. Understanding the unique barriers to effective diabetes management in Latino communities—including language, cultural differences, income and education levels, health insurance coverage, and more—is important, as is finding a good diabetes doctor or educator who can help you gain the knowledge you need to manage your blood sugar with good results.

CHAPTER 2

Understanding Body Fat, Fitness, and Diabetes

As a Latino, you may perceive obesity differently from people belonging to other cultures, and you may even believe that being overweight is a sign of being healthy. Latina mothers have long taken it as a compliment when someone calls their child *gordito* because a chubby baby is considered to be strong and healthy. But a chubby child, especially of Latino descent, is likely to suffer from type 2 diabetes, high blood pressure, and high cholesterol at an early age. Moreover, if you have become Americanized, you may have lost some of the healthier, traditional habits of many Latinos.

Being Latino and having close family members with diabetes increases your risk of developing it, especially if you are overweight or obese. However, having a family history does not mandate that you will get diabetes, nor does carrying extra body fat, which is not necessarily a direct cause as once thought. Where you carry your excess fat—if it's stored in your abdomen as a type called visceral fat (intra-abdominal fat)—does affect your risk, as explained in Chapter 1. But is it correct to blame your genes and body fat for your diabetes? We'll try to answer this question and give you some alternate explanations and solutions, along with more information about the downside of dieting, the importance of physical fitness, and how to improve your body's insulin action to prevent and control diabetes.

Getting diabetes is not all due to being Latino

You can't entirely blame your diabetes on your "bad" genes or some other uncontrollable factor. For example, the Pima Native Americans of Arizona have an extremely high incidence of obesity, insulin resistance (prediabetes), and type 2 diabetes. Given that more than half of all Pima adults thirty-five and older develop type 2 diabetes, many researchers had previously concluded that most Pimas are genetically doomed to gain excessive amounts of body weight and develop this disease.

Environmental factors may actually be more important than genes. Researchers recently found another group of Pimas, from whom the Arizona group apparently descended, living in Sonora, Mexico (technically making them Latinos). Despite their common gene pool, the two groups differ dramatically in their levels of body fat and incidence of diabetes. The Americanized Arizona Pimas live like most of us, eating highly refined, nutrient-poor foods and too many calories; moreover, they have adopted the sedentary lifestyle that exemplifies Americans today. By contrast, the Mexican Pimas are physically active farmers, eating a traditional diet of natural foods such as wheat, squash, beans, cactus buds, squawfish, and jackrabbit, which they grow or catch themselves. Would you be surprised to learn that while more than 50 percent of the adult Pimas living in the United States develop type 2 diabetes, their Mexican "cousins" remain diabetes-free and lean—in spite of sharing the same genes? This example shows you the power that lifestyle choices have in determining your diabetes fate.

It's not all due to being overweight or obese either

Excess body fat is a hot topic in the news, and weight loss is the focus of popular reality TV shows like *The Biggest Loser*. In the United States, over 30 percent of adults, 15.5 percent of adolescents (ages 12–19), and 15.3 percent of children (ages 6–11) are obese, and about 65 percent of adults are considered overweight. Obesity among children has almost tripled in the past two decades, and unfortunately Latino children have been particularly affected—and at younger ages.

Do you need to lose all of your excess fat to be healthy? Or would it help to lose just some of it? Currently, the worldwide type 2 diabetes epidemic is closely paralleling an increase in body fat around the world, and about 90 percent of newly diagnosed diabetic individuals are either overweight or obese. With the close association between the two epidemics, it is not surprising that extra fat gets blamed for type 2 diabetes and associated health problems. In the past decade, researchers held obesity directly responsible for hyperinsulinemia (elevated levels of insulin in the blood) and glucose intolerance (your body's inability to handle glucose and other carbohydrates without an excessive rise in blood sugars), both of which are associated with insulin resistance and prediabetes. In addition, obesity has been blamed for a higher incidence of congestive heart failure and heart disease, gallstones, gout, arthritis, sleep apnea, certain types of cancer (endometrial, breast, prostate, and colon), infertility and menstrual irregularities in women, and psychological disorders.

Before jumping to any conclusions, you need to consider whether the coexistence of these health problems with excess body fat proves that fat is the cause of these diseases or is actually a symptom. Fat cells (adipocytes) were until recently thought to be dormant storage depots of fat, but we now know that fat cells actually communicate with other parts of your body by releasing hormones like leptin and adiponectin that affect food intake, fat storage, and more. While we're still learning more about these fat-related hormones, we do know that leptin may have direct effects on your liver's storage of glucose, which may largely determine whether or not someone who is obese will develop diabetes or not.

While excess body fat is not harmless, the purported health benefits of substantial weight loss have likely been exaggerated. Excess body fat is more appropriately considered a symptom of diabetes, or a contributor to its development, rather than its sole cause. In laboratory tests isolated fat cells respond normally to insulin even when they come from insulin-resistant donors. Excess body fat can't be the sole problem if the same fat cells that are insulin resistant in a person's body are perfectly receptive to insulin when removed from the body and tested in a lab.

What's likely is that a sedentary lifestyle contributes more to insulin resistance and diabetes onset than body fat. Both your fat and muscle cells become more responsive to insulin when you do regular aerobic exercise—whether you lose any weight or not—even though both types of cells can contribute heavily to insulin resistance. You'll read more about how to enhance your body's insulin action later in this chapter.

What role does your body shape play?

Remember that visceral (intra-abdominal) body fat mentioned at the beginning of this chapter? As already noted, all body fat is not harmful. But where you store your excess fat may have some importance, regardless of how much you have. Recent studies have shown that people who store more fat subcutaneously—in fat cells right under the surface of the skin—are actually more insulin sensitive and better off, metabolically speaking, than those who store fat within the abdominal cavity.

Unfortunately, body fat patterning is genetically predetermined, meaning that you can control the total amount of fat you store but not where you store it. This patterning is reflected in your waist-to-hip ratio (WHR). To determine your WHR, first measure your waist as the circumference (in inches or centimeters) even with your belly button, and then take your hip measurements around the widest part of your buttocks. Due to the anatomical differences between men and women, optimal values for WHR differ by sex, although a ratio of less than or equal to 0.9 reduces metabolic and diabetes risk for men, while 0.8 is the cutoff for women. For either sex, a WHR greater than 1.0 places you in the danger zone for developing health problems.

A high WHR, or abdominal obesity (an apple body shape more typical in men), results when a greater amount of metabolically active visceral fat is stored deep within the abdominal cavity, in and around your internal organs. This fat may be easier to gain and lose, but it has a stronger association with insulin resistance, type 2 diabetes, high blood pressure, and heart disease. Being pear-shaped (heavier around the hips and thighs) is more common in women and corresponds to a reduced risk of having diabetes. It's far better to be a pear than an apple, although you don't have much say about which one you are.

Nowadays, relying on the WHR to assess diabetes risk is considered less effective than just measuring your waist circumference. For men at least, the bigger their waist, the greater their risk of developing type 2 diabetes. Men with waists that are 37.9 to 39.8

inches in circumference, for example, have a risk of developing diabetes that is five times greater than men whose waists are 29 to 34 inches, likely due to increased amounts of stored visceral fat. Women's waists should be less than 34.7 inches to minimize their diabetes risk.

If not in fat cells, where else do excess calories get stored?

Did you know that your body stores fat from excess calories in places other than fat cells? Both your muscles and your liver store extra fat as you get heavier. More fat storage in your muscles may decrease the uptake of blood glucose (removal of glucose from your blood into muscle cells) into those areas, making them more resistant to insulin if you don't exercise regularly. Given that your muscles are responsible for the majority of blood glucose uptake and use in response to insulin, becoming insulin resistant in muscles has a substantial impact on your blood sugar. Regular exercisers, paradoxically, can store more fat in their muscles without experiencing insulin resistance, suggesting that the total amount of fat stored in your muscles may not be the critical component but rather the way muscles respond to insulin.

The greater release of insulin that results from eating excessive amounts of carbohydrates may cause you to gain body fat because carbohydrates are usually converted into and stored as fat when you are sedentary. If you store fat just in fat cells (particularly in the ones under the skin), you probably will not have as many health problems compared to when your body has to resort to putting it elsewhere. For example, storing extra fat in your liver may contribute to low-level inflammation throughout your body, which can lead to the development of insulin resistance, diabetes, heart disease, and other metabolic disorders. Therefore your liver (and whether it stores excess fat) may prove to be a crucial link between weight gain and the development of prediabetes and type 2 diabetes.

An insulin-resistant liver may account for elevated blood fats and cholesterol levels that contribute to the development of heart disease, including reductions in HDL cholesterol, the good type of cholesterol. You can compound the problem by eating foods that contribute to your liver's insulin resistance, including those high in refined carbohydrates and processed foods. You have the power to lower your body's inflammation and improve your metabolic health with lifestyle changes that will be discussed in the chapters that follow.

Why going on a diet isn't the best solution for body weight or health

In Latino communities, being overweight is not the big emotional or social issue that it is in many others. An overweight baby is often viewed as healthy, rather than as a child who is likely to have issues with his weight and health throughout his lifetime. Nevertheless, Hispanic communities are beginning to realize that excess body weight can have undesirable health effects.

To improve your health, you don't have to reach some unrealistically low body weight. In fact, losing just ten pounds improves your insulin action, lowers your systemic inflammation, enhances your good cholesterol and lowers the bad, improves your metabolic efficiency, and dramatically reduces your diabetes risk. Going on a diet to lose weight, however, is not the best long-term solution to managing your body weight or reducing your diabetes risk. Why? Dieting does not work for most people. It becomes progressively harder to lose weight the longer you stay on a diet (thus making it harder for you to stay motivated to follow it); consequently, many people give up after a while.

However, the real problem with dieting is that you are not likely to keep off any weight that you do lose. As many as nine out of ten dieters who have successfully lost weight ultimately regain the pounds they struggled to lose. If you go back to eating the same foods after your diet ends that you ate before, you will typically rebound by taking in excessive calories, particularly in the form of extra fat that quickly returns you to your prediet weight. In fact, most people gain back even more than they lost, regardless of the diet they followed. A greater percentage of the weight you regain is usually body fat, ultimately making your body fat higher than if you had never lost any weight.

While your body's set point—or what you normally weigh—can change gradually over your lifetime, it remains the same over the relatively short time frame of a diet, unless you make permanent lifestyle changes. So, if you have to choose between dieting and becoming more physically active to lose weight, always choose the latter. When you experience large fluctuations in body weight over time, you're likely to be less healthy than people who never lost weight in the first place. Women whose body weight goes up and down may actually have a greater risk of developing heart disease.

If you lose weight, keep it off

If you are one of the fortunate people who have kept off the weight you lost, congratulations. If not, you may benefit from learning how others have done it. The National Weight Control Registry has tracked individuals who have lost at least thirty pounds and kept the weight off for at least a year. (Keeping it off more than six months is very uncommon even among successful dieters.) It doesn't appear to make any difference what method or weight loss plan they use to lose weight; their food choices range from a conventional lower-calorie, moderate-carbohydrate diets like Weight Watchers and Jenny Craig to low-carb ones like Atkins and South Beach.

Most important is the two lifestyle habits that almost all of them adopt: They continue to be conscientious about what they eat (more healthful food in appropriate portions) and exercise almost daily, expending about 2,000 calories a week in physical activity. In addition, most continue to eat a healthy breakfast. Only a minority of them (17 percent) consume a low-carbohydrate diet to control their weight, regardless of what diet they followed to lose the extra pounds. On average, their diets have about 50 percent of calories coming from carbohydrates, 30 percent from fat, and the remainder (about 20 percent) from protein. In comparison, those who regain the most weight have higher calorie intake, eat more fast foods and fat, and have lower levels of physical activity.

Is it possible to keep the weight from coming back on? Most Americans have little success in preventing the weight gain that typically comes with getting older. We strongly advocate that you simply get physically active and don't worry about maintaining a specific weight. Despite the hundreds of thousands of calories that you typically eat in the course of a year, your body has the innate ability to match food intake with calorie expenditure and is capable of maintaining your body weight within a pound or two. Likely, the biggest contributor to weight gain in Latinos today is expending too few calories through physical activity.

You can also prevent or reverse weight gain over time by making small changes in your daily habits. A pound of fat equals about 3,500 calories, so if you eat just fifty more calories than you use each day (the equivalent of less than a quarter cup of cooked rice, white or brown), your total weight gain can be just five pounds of body fat in a year. If you cut back by fifty calories a day—by leaving a few bites uneaten at each meal or skipping a small treat—and combine that with expending an extra fifty calories a day by doing some extra walking, stretching, or other easy activity, you can lose ten pounds of body fat in a year.

Walking may prevent diabetes

If you have a dog that demands daily walking, you may be less likely to develop diabetes because research has shown that type 2 diabetes may actually be preventable with regular walking combined with other minor lifestyle improvements. For example, the Diabetes Prevention Program (DPP) studied 3,234 overweight American adults with impaired glucose tolerance (diagnosed with an oral glucose tolerance test) at high risk for diabetes, almost half of whom were from high-risk ethnic groups like Latinos. Participants in the lifestyle arm of the study followed a lower fat diet and increased their exercise to include 150 minutes per week of a moderately intense activity (most did brisk walking) spread out over at least three days. After just three years, people who had made these improvements in their daily habits had reduced their average risk of developing diabetes by 58 percent, despite their high risk of developing diabetes. The preventive benefits were even more pronounced among ethnic groups and older individuals, the people most often affected by diabetes.

Walking appeared to be enough to prevent diabetes, and participants who walked two and a half hours or more a week had a 63 to 69 percent lower risk of developing diabetes. Admittedly, the DPP study did not test the role of regular physical activity without simultaneous changes in diet and body weight, but weight loss was minimal; on average, participants lost about 7 percent of their body weight, equivalent to just fourteen pounds for a two hundred pound person or twenty-one pounds for a three hundred pound one. Your genes also influence how effective lifestyle changes are in preventing diabetes, with some people responding to exercise, others to weight loss, and the remainder to dietary changes. A follow-up analysis of this study's results found that weight loss was important—participants' risk of diabetes decreased by 16 percent for each kilogram (2.2 pounds) they lost. But only the individuals who continued to exercise regularly maintained their weight loss and kept their risk of diabetes lower.

Other studies have shown amazingly similar results despite being conducted in countries with high rates of diabetes, such as Finland and China. The Finnish Diabetes Prevention Study also found a 58 percent reduction in diabetes risk with lifestyle improvements, including regular walking. Moreover, a follow-up to that study found that people eating a low-fat, high-fiber diet lost more weight and kept it off longer and that this intervention itself led to sustained lifestyle changes, resulting in a lower risk of type 2 diabetes even after lifestyle counseling (offered through the study) was stopped. A twenty-year follow-up to the China study found that group-based lifestyle interventions, such as organized walking programs, can prevent or delay the onset of diabetes for up to fourteen years afterward.

JOSÉ CORTEZ
A champion for diabetes prevention in the Latino community

Some members of the Latino community have chosen to help lead the way in educating others and preventing the onset of diabetes. José Cortez, for example, is a public relations manager at a community development corporation based in Phoenix, Arizona, called Chicanos por La Causa. He is also a member of the National Diabetes Education Program's Prevengamos diabetes tipo 2. Paso a paso (Small Steps, Big Rewards

Team to Fight Diabetes). A father of six in his late fifties, José strives to demonstrate that type 2 diabetes can be prevented in the Latino community.

"Over ten years ago, I started taking steps to get healthy. I was forty-six years old, feeling out of shape and older than my age," he recalls. "Around this time, I began learning about different health risks prevalent within the Latino community. While doing this research, I learned about the diabetes epidemic and the health risks associated with people in my community and of my age." His wife is a Pima Native American, and about half of her tribe had already been diagnosed with diabetes. He continues, "I realized that not only were my wife and I at risk for type 2 diabetes, but our children were also. I had to improve the health of my family and community because I didn't want this deadly disease or anyone else in my family to suffer from it."

To begin having a better lifestyle, José made a commitment to hike a local mountain each morning. Taking the time to do so for him was a small price to pay given how much better he started to feel physically and mentally. "I was relaxed at work and dealt with stressful situations more effectively. I also became increasingly aware of my eating habits and began making healthier choices." He claims that this simple routine of hiking every day changed his life—and his outlook on life.

José also took it upon himself to show his coworkers how to become more physically active after he noticed that many of them were so unfit that they had difficulty just walking around the block. And these were people working at a firm responsible for improving the quality of life for the Latinos in Phoenix! He says, "I began a workplace health and wellness program to help my colleagues get moving. I used my research about diabetes in our community and my personal experiences with physical activity and eating well to develop the program." His goal is to make the Latino community aware of its predisposition to diabetes, starting with his coworkers. He realizes that nothing happens overnight, but he firmly believes that as a community, he and others can begin to turn the tide back on the diabetes epidemic by getting moving and taking small steps in that direction.

How did we become so physically inactive?

The best way to avoid weight gain in the first place is to exercise regularly. A recent study concluded that young Americans are becoming overweight mainly because they don't move around enough, and the same is true for adults. There are many other reasons why becoming physically active is more than worth the effort. The more sedentary you are, the greater your risk of dying prematurely from myriad causes. Even more important, though, is your increased chance of not feeling good while you are alive. Nevertheless, nearly half of all American adults are not active, while 70 percent fail to meet the recommended thirty minutes of exercise a day most days of the week. Ask yourself if you really want to spend the last twenty years of your life impaired by diabetic complications when you can improve your quality of life with diabetes and prevent most health problems by becoming more fit.

Why are people so inactive nowadays? Unlike our Mexican Pima cousins, for the most part we have become the modern-day hunter-gatherers who no longer hunt our food or grow it ourselves. In the past half century, Americans have experienced a rise in sedentary, leisure-time pursuits unparalleled in human history. Labor-saving devices like dishwashers, remote controls, and personal computers have left most people sitting more than ever. You can watch hundreds of channels on your TV, shop on the Internet without ever leaving your chair, and communicate with everyone via cell phones and email.

Although sitting around is generally unhealthy, TV watching appears to be especially detrimental because you expend less energy watching TV than engaging in other sedentary activities, such as playing board games or reading. It's almost like being asleep. If your kids watch a lot of TV, they're more likely to have bad eating habits, such as munching on unhealthy, high-calorie snacks while watching the many junk food commercials targeting youth (if you choose to buy those snacks for them, that is). The negative effects of excess TV time apparently last through adulthood as well. The amount of time you spent watching TV during your childhood and adolescence is also directly associated with your risk of high cholesterol, diabetes, poor fitness, smoking, and obesity as an adult. In short, we have become a society of overweight, sedentary people.

Diet also plays a dramatic role in the poor physical condition of most Americans, not just Hispanics. Not only have portion sizes increased during the past several decades, but we have also become entrenched in a fast food mentality. We expect and demand greater selections of fast food restaurants and low-nutrition, prepackaged food ready for consumption in super-size "bargain" portions. And most of the smaller, hundred-calorie packs are not the best type of snacks for diabetes prevention and control and optimal health. You can use a drive-though and pick up your food without even getting out of your car. It's a vicious cycle because you will likely move around less after gaining excess weight from poor food choices, and then being more sedentary causes you to gain more weight, and so on. Despite the proven and publicized health benefits of physical activity, the vast majority of us remain sedentary, unfit, and overweight.

Insulin resistance in type 2 diabetes and prediabetes

The latest research links a lack of physical activity directly to defects in the action of insulin primarily at the level of your muscle and fat cells. Think of muscle as a "glucose sink" (or a place like a warehouse) to store the carbohydrates that you eat and don't use right away. When you exercise regularly, you use up your muscle glycogen (the

---

Factors That Can Improve Insulin Action in Muscles

- Regular aerobic and resistance exercise
- Muscle mass gain
- Loss of body fat, particularly visceral fat and extra fat stored in the liver
- Improved blood glucose control
- Reduced levels of circulating free fatty acids (one type of fat in blood)
- Reduction in low-level, systemic inflammation
- More effective action of leptin (an adipose hormone), causing reduced food intake
- Reduction in mental (anxiety, depression) and/or physical (e.g., illness) stressors
- Decrease in circulating levels of cortisol
- Increased testosterone levels in men
- Intake of more dietary fiber, less saturated and trans fat, and fewer highly refined foods
- Daily consumption of a healthy breakfast
- Lower caffeine intake
- Adequate sleep (seven to eight hours a night for most adults)
- Effective treatment of sleep apnea
- Use of insulin-sensitizing medications

---

form of blood glucose stored in the muscles) and have room to put carbohydrates back in after you eat. If the glycogen stores are already full because you have consumed too many carbohydrates and exercised too little, your muscles fail to respond to the insulin released by your pancreas when you eat, making you more insulin resistant, which likely is combined with or caused by systemic inflammation (both of which are reversible by exercise).

Moreover, the carbohydrates you eat end up spiking your blood sugar, which causes the release of more insulin and ultimately the storage of more fat in adipose (and likely liver) cells around your body. Fat cells remain responsive to insulin even when your muscle cells become resistant, and much of your excess blood glucose can be converted into storage fat. If your body releases a large amount of insulin in response to rice or other carbohydrates you eat, you'll probably benefit from a low-carb diet, especially if you're trying to lose weight or improve insulin action in your muscles. Many other factors can improve your body's insulin sensitivity and consequently reverse prediabetes or improve diabetes control.

Thus you can reverse prediabetes or better manage your diabetes simply by implementing positive changes in your exercise and dietary habits. The next two chapters will explain in more detail what changes are most important and how to implement them into your lifestyle.

CHAPTER 2: *En pocas palabras*

Latinos can't blame their genes entirely for causing diabetes, nor is being overweight the sole culprit. Where your body stores fat may influence the development of diabetes, though, and fat stored inside your abdomen and in other cells around your body (e.g., muscle and liver) appears to be most harmful. Dieting is not necessarily the answer to preventing or reversing diabetes, although some weight loss can have a positive effect. Among the factors that can impact your body's insulin action and risk of diabetes, being physically active ranks high in importance, even if your activity is walking the dog.

CHAPTER 3

Going Beyond the
Latino Diet

If you are of Latino descent, your diet is more likely than your body weight to dictate whether you suffer from type 2 diabetes, high blood pressure, and high cholesterol. It is imperative that Latinos (children and adults) eat a healthy diet that helps prevent these problems. In this chapter, you will learn how to incorporate a Latino diet (particularly its flavors and ingredients) into a healthy and diabetes-controlling menu when you include more traditional foods and fewer refined ones.

What do Latinos eat?

There is no typical Latino food, but rather many dishes that originated in the blend of influences from Native American, African, Asian, Indian, Caribbean, European, and other cuisines. Also, the "typical" cuisine varies from country to country, and even single dishes vary by region within a country. Some examples of foods are maize-based dishes (e.g., tortillas, tamales, tacos, *tortas, tlacoyos, tlayudas,* and *pupusas*), meat-based ones containing chicken, beef, fish, or lamb; various salsas and condiments like guacamole and pico de gallo, and spices that vary by country. Common beverages include *mate, Pisco Sour, horchata, chicha, atole, cacao,* and *agua fresca.* As in American cuisine, desserts are ubiquitous in Latino cooking; some of the more favored ones are very sweet, such as *dulce de leche, alfajor, arroz con leche, tres leches* cake, *Teja,* and flan. In certain cuisines, rice is also common, along with legumes (beans).

The cuisine reflects each country's agricultural strengths and weaknesses based on geography. Most Americans' concept of Latino cuisine is Mexican food, but authentic Mexican cuisine hardly resembles the Tex-Mex version found in the United States. Traditional cuisines from Mexico and Central America use primarily grains and fruits and vegetables, complemented with meat from small animals like ducks, chickens, and turkeys—and even insects. Costa Ricans, however, eat more fresh fruits and vegetables, rice, black beans, corn tortillas, white cheese (a nonprocessed cheese made from adding salt to milk in production), and *picadillos* (made with ground beef). Some coastal countries like Honduras and Chile include more seafood and shellfish in their cooking, while others have access to more tropical fruits and coconuts. Corn is a staple in many of them, though, along with varying types of rice. Argentina, by contrast, is a major producer of meat (especially beef), wheat, corn, milk, beans, and soybeans. Red meat is a common part of the Argentine diet. Due to the large number of Argentines of Italian ancestry, pizza and pasta are also very popular, and they have adopted food traditions from other countries, including English afternoon tea.

Latino-style eating is not necessarily good for diabetes control

In many Hispanic countries, a light meal is served for breakfast, such as eggs, pastries (e.g., *pan dulce*, or sweet bread), coffee, and milk, or leftovers from the day before. While it is well acknowledged in the diabetes world that breakfast is an important meal to reduce insulin resistance, the type of breakfast you eat can also influence how your body responds. Generally, your morning meal should include minimal amounts of refined carbohydrates that can raise blood sugar rapidly at that time of day; neither pastries nor pan dulce is a good choice, and you would do best to avoid other sugar-sweetened foods. It's much better to start the day with high-quality protein foods and a small amount of fresh fruit.

For Latinos, lunch usually is the main meal of the day. In some Hispanic countries, adult family members and children come home from work or school for about two hours to be together for this meal, which often includes a siesta taken after lunch. In the early evening, a light snack of coffee and rolls or sandwiches is served informally or just for the youngsters in the family. The last meal of the day is a small supper that is often eaten as late as 9:00 P.M. Eating the largest meal of the day at lunch usually leads to less weight gain than overeating calories late in the evening, as many Americans do. Latinos living in the United States tend to adopt the American three-meal system, but midday and evening meals remain important family or social events, with time to linger over coffee or an after-dinner drink. Hispanics who maintain their original diet of mostly low-calorie and low-fat foods and minimally processed fruits and vegetables have better health outcomes than those who become acculturated to the typical American way of eating.

Unfortunately, moderate food intake is not traditionally part of Hispanic cultures. Eating is the main focus of almost all Latino social activities (as it is in many other cultures as well) and refusing to eat, even when eating more would be excessive, is considered disrespectful. Usually when additional servings of food are offered, we Latinos tend to accept only after the second or third time. Although excessive consumption of food can lead to weight gain or obesity, as a Latino, you may have a different concept of thinness than others, particularly white Americans. Latinos have deep-seated cultural assumptions about healthy living and healthy appearance, and being overweight as a child and even into adulthood may be considered a sign of health and higher socioeconomic status, as we mentioned previously.

Why the type of carbohydrate matters

Can you have a healthy diet and remain true to your Latino cuisine? It is entirely possible as long as you keep a few concepts in mind. A balanced meal plan, according to the latest dietary recommendations, contains 45 to 65 percent of calories from carbohydrates, 20 to 35 percent of calories from fat, and 10 to 35 percent from protein. However, a recent research study strongly suggests that it is not the amount of carbohydrates you eat that makes you gain weight as much as the type. Among the 572 adults in that study, those who ate more refined grains (e.g., white rice), starchy vegetables (e.g., white potatoes), white flour products, and other low-nutrition carbohydrates were significantly heavier than those who ate foods containing healthier whole grains, nonstarchy vegetables, and nuts and seeds. Body fat does not break down when your insulin levels are high, which happens when you eat processed or refined carbohydrates and you are insulin resistant. Thus limiting your intake of carbohydrates that require either greater release or doses of insulin will make it easier for you to lose weight, if that is your goal.

A lower-carbohydrate diet, in addition to lowering your blood lipids and your blood glucose, will also help you keep the weight off. Body weight is generally higher in people who consume carbohydrate-rich foods that are rapidly absorbed (i.e., those with a greater effect on blood sugar, as we will explain later in this chapter) and cause spikes in blood glucose. Since your fat cells remain responsive to insulin, your blood sugars may be running high, but you'll be gaining fat weight at the same time. It's virtually impossible to lose body fat when your insulin levels are high. In any case, you will likely benefit from limiting your intake of refined carbohydrates for many reasons, weight management being just one of them.

For optimal health, you should focus on eating an anti-inflammatory diet, one that reduces compounds in your blood (e.g., C-reactive peptide) that are indicative of low-level, systemic inflammation. An inflammatory diet is one laden with highly processed, calorie-dense, nutrient-depleted foods like french fries and other fast foods that most Americans—Latinos included—currently eat. This type of diet frequently leads to exaggerated spikes in blood glucose levels after meals. These spikes cause oxidative stress, leading to systemic inflammation, which contributes to insulin resistance, heart disease, and other health problems, particularly when the foods you eat are lacking in antioxidants and other essential nutrients that can help combat this damage.

To prevent blood glucose spikes after meals, focus on eating minimally processed, high-fiber, plant-based foods—most fruits and vegetables, whole grains, legumes, nuts, lean protein sources (like egg whites and whey protein), vinegar, fish oil, tea, and cinnamon. An anti-inflammatory diet can also include traditional Latino foods like papayas, corn tortillas, and avocados. Avoid highly processed foods and beverages, particularly ones containing high-fructose corn syrup, sugar, white flour, or trans fats. It also helps to limit your portions to moderate amounts and exercise regularly.

Good dietary guidelines for diabetes control

The American Diabetes Association no longer advocates a specific diet for people with diabetes, although they have done so in the past. The esteemed Joslin Diabetes Center in Boston recently released its own dietary and exercise guidelines for overweight people with either type 2 diabetes or prediabetes. Joslin's guidelines (available at www.joslin.org/Files/Nutrition_Guideline_Graded.pdf) provide clear and easy-to-follow recommendations to improve insulin sensitivity and cardiovascular health while reducing body fat.

The Joslin Center's diabetes researchers and experts recommend that about 40 percent of your daily calories come from carbohydrates, 20 to 30 percent from protein (except if you have known kidney problems), and 30 to 35 percent from fat (mostly mono- and polyunsaturated fats), along with a minimum of 20 to 35 grams of fiber (with a goal of 50 grams, if you can tolerate that much).

The actual composition of carbohydrate, fat, and protein you consume is less important than the effect that individual foods have on your blood glucose levels, though. For weight loss, the Joslin researchers advocate reducing daily caloric intake by 250 to 500 calories a day to allow a gradual weight loss of no more than one pound every one to two weeks. Minimally, women should consume no less than 1,000 to 1,200 calories per day versus 1,200 to 1,600 for men. Finally, they recommend a target of sixty to ninety minutes of moderate-intensity physical activity, including cardiovascular, stretching, and resistance activities, most days of the week, with at least 150 to 175 minutes weekly.

Balanced meal plans are undeniably the best ones to follow over the long term, whether you have diabetes or not. Although no foods are completely forbidden in the Joslin plan, researchers suggest that you consume fewer carbohydrates with higher glycemic effect, which means limiting your intake of refined carbohydrates or processed grains and starchy foods like pasta, white bread, low-fiber cereal, and white potatoes. Their endorsement of a 40 percent carbohydrate diet likely stems from the fact that most Americans are not likely to remove enough refined carbohydrates from their diet to effectively moderate the glycemic effect of eating more of them. If you emphasize healthier sources, you will not need to cut all carbohydrates out of your diet, likewise with fats and proteins, as long as you choose better fats and leaner sources of protein. These guidelines are the most powerfully health-promoting ones ever endorsed for prevention and control of type 2 diabetes.

Foods in their natural state are always best

While foods are being processed (as when whole wheat is made into white flour, bleached or unbleached), numerous nutrients are stripped out and only a select few are added back in by manufacturers. The result is that processed foods are far less nutritious than foods in a more natural state. Nutrients in foods work best the way they grew, and often the synergy of the nutrients in food is as vital as the individual nutrients themselves.

Fruits and vegetables in their natural state are particularly rich in compounds called phytochemicals (phytonutrients), which are found in plants and have disease-fighting and health-promoting powers; some examples are capsaicin, lycopene, lutein, quercetin, saponins, and terpenes. Most can't be bought in supplement form, nor would you really want to consume them without the benefits of the bioactive substances in whole foods. Certain foods containing phytonutrients may one day cure diabetes. It was recently discovered that tart cherries increase insulin production in beta cells by 50 percent due to their anthocyanin, which contributes to the fruit's bright red color. This phytonutrient can also be found in other bright red, blue, and purple produce—such as red grapes, strawberries, and blueberries—as well as in wine, cider, and tea.

Americans have gotten into the bad habit of eating foods that are colorless, including white bread, white rice, white potatoes, white sugar, and white (iceberg) lettuce, whereas you need to choose foods from a minimum of four color groups daily: red, orange-yellow, green, and blue-purple. The phytonutrients in each color group vary with the pigment. For example, red foods like tomatoes and tomato products contain lycopene, which may prevent prostate cancer in men; the carotenoids in orange-yellow foods may reduce your risk of heart disease; green foods like broccoli contain sulforaphane, a cancer fighter; and blueberries, in the last color group, contain nearly one hundred different known phytonutrients, making them the top-ranked food in terms of antioxidants and disease-fighting power.

In general, darker-colored foods have more phytonutrients. The majority of these compounds are found in the dark outer coatings that contain the antioxidants plants use to protect themselves from oxidative damage by the sun's ultraviolet rays. Legumes illustrate this concept well: Black beans are highest in antioxidants (flavonoids), followed by the red, brown, yellow, and white varieties, in decreasing amounts. Red and purple grapes also contain more of these compounds than green ones.

Since the majority of diabetic complications are also likely related to unchecked oxidative stress in various tissues and organs, eating foods containing more antioxidant power may mitigate the negative impact of elevated blood glucose. In addition to blueberries, other potent fruits to include in your diet are strawberries, raspberries, oranges, mangoes, grapefruit (particularly pink), kiwi, avocados, concord grapes, cherries, and plums. Also, eat more tomatoes, broccoli, red bell peppers, sweet potatoes (the vegetable highest in vitamins A and C, folate, iron, copper, calcium, and fiber), carrots (second best), winter squash, kale, spinach, purple cabbage, and eggplant. You'll also be happy to hear that dark chocolate and cocoa, red wine, green and black tea, and coffee also have large amounts of antioxidants, but moderate your consumption of dark chocolate and wine to avoid taking in too many calories and limit your coffee intake because caffeine can decrease insulin action. In addition to eating them in natural foods, you can also take supplements containing antioxidants, which are currently popular because of their purported ability to slow aging caused by cumulative oxidative damage in the body; some of these supplements are discussed in more detail in the following chapter.

Tips for Preparing Healthier Meals

- Cook with olive or canola oil. Go easy on the oil (or use a cooking spray) and avoid frying foods.
- Use lean cuts of meat, including beef with all visible fat removed; skinless chicken and turkey breast; lean ground beef, chicken, or turkey; tofu and soy protein.
- Bake, broil, poach, or grill meat, fish, and chicken rather than frying them.
- Buy lower-fat (and sugar-free, whenever possible) varieties of dairy products, including milk, cheese, sour cream, yogurt, and ice cream.
- Eat veggies raw, steamed, microwaved, or grilled, using only light seasonings or spicy peppers rather than drenching them with creamy, cheesy, or buttery sauces.

- Avoid boiling vegetables in water to prevent the loss of key vitamins and minerals into the liquid (or drink the "mineralized" water too).
- Use mainly fresh or frozen vegetables and fruits; canned ones typically contain added salt and/or sugar. If you must, use only canned fruit packed in its own juices.
- Keep fresh vegetables like baby carrots, broccoli, peppers, or cauliflower handy for snacks, and eat them with a healthy dip like hummus (chickpeas and sesame tahini) and fat-free or olive oil-based dressings.
- Snack on whole fruits instead of manufactured products containing fruit, and keep a variety of fruits—such as grapes, apples, oranges, bananas, and seasonal fruit—on hand for healthy snacks (but watch how many carbohydrates you are eating).
- If you drink fruit juice, use only the 100 percent juice varieties and limit yourself to no more than four ounces at a time; avoid juices with high fructose corn syrup as a main ingredient.
- On salads, use balsamic vinegar, reduced-calorie, or fat-free dressings. Go easy on the amount that you use, keeping in mind that dressings containing olive oil are still high in calories, while fat-free varieties often have added sugar or high-fructose corn syrup.
- Add cut-up vegetables to canned beans, soups, or omelets to increase their nutrient value, water content, and fiber.
- Buy only bread products that list whole wheat as the first ingredient on the food label, and use other whole grain products whenever possible (while limiting your total intake).
- Add extra fiber into recipes for baked goods, casseroles, and soups by spooning in a few tablespoons of oat bran, wheat bran, or milled flax seed when you prepare them.
- For baked goods, add only one-half to two-thirds of the sugar called for by the recipe and use healthier margarines (also reducing the amount).

Why is fiber intake so important?

"Fiber" is a collective term for all indigestible polysaccharides (a type of complex carbohydrate), including the natural ones in foods and others that are extracted or isolated from foods or made synthetically (e.g., Metamucil). Soluble fiber—found in oatmeal, legumes, seeds, fruits (such as apples, bananas, citrus fruits), and vegetables— dissolves in water, is partially metabolized in the large intestine by friendly bacteria, and plays a major role in removing cholesterol from the body. An insoluble form of fiber is found in vegetables like carrots, celery, and the skins of corn kernels; fruit peels, cores, and seeds; brown rice; and whole grains, or the outer membranes of wheat kernels. This fiber, acting as roughage, passes through your digestive system without being fully digested and ensures regular bowel movements. It's a good idea to drink an extra glass or two of water during the day to go along with your extra fiber.

Although the low-carb craze has resulted in many new products with added fiber (including pasta and tortilla shells), generally the more refined a product is, the less fiber it is likely to contain. To find out the fiber content of any food, either read its nutrition label (if it comes in a box or package) or, for produce or natural foods, look up fiber information on nutrition-related websites. A reasonable fiber goal is a minimum of 12.5 grams per 1,000 calories that you eat daily. Alternatively, instead of trying to eat a certain amount, you can focus on eating more whole grains, fruits, vegetables, and legumes to increase your fiber intake.

There are many health-related reasons to eat more fiber. A high-fiber diet may help reduce your chances of developing heart disease, diabetes, obesity, strokes, colorectal and other types of cancer, diverticulosis, and hemorrhoids. If you are at high risk of developing type 2 diabetes, a diet high in fiber enhances your insulin sensitivity. A recent study showed that a portion-controlled, low-glycemic diet containing Mexican-style foods (such as pinto beans, whole wheat bread, and low-glycemic fruits) can improve glucose levels in obese people with type 2 diabetes due largely to its low glycemic effect and high fiber content. Fiber also aids in portion control because it generally slows down the rate at which food empties from your stomach, makes you feel full longer, and helps prevent excessive eating and weight gain.

Foods that are higher in fiber are also, on the whole, lower in added sugars, fat, and calories. As noted, the best strategy to control your diabetes is not to completely eliminate carbohydrates but rather to eat higher-fiber ones. If you eat a low-fiber food like a candy bar, you will likely still feel hungry afterward despite an excessive intake of calories and a spike in blood glucose. If you eat a high-fiber, medium-size apple along with a small handful of nuts or a chunk of low-fat cheese instead, it will take you longer to eat and, in the end, you will feel satiated by fewer calories while achieving better blood sugar control.

What types of fat are good?

Not every type of fat is bad for you, but a high intake of saturated and trans fats can contribute to the development of insulin resistance as much as an excess intake of sugars and refined carbohydrates. Diabetes also usually results in unhealthy changes in your blood fats. Elevated levels of triglycerides (mainly from dietary fat, but also formed in your body when you eat highly refined carbohydrates) and bad types of cholesterol play a major role in stimulating the inflammatory process leading to the development of cardiovascular disease common to diabetes.

Saturated and trans fats found in dairy products, meat, hydrogenated oils, and highly processed foods increase your insulin resistance and make it harder to keep blood sugar and cholesterol levels under control. For example, eating even one fast food meal high in saturated fat can interrupt the normal flow of blood through your arteries and veins for hours afterward and make your body's response to insulin sluggish as well. Conversely, if you eat a high-fat breakfast that contains mostly a good fat like olive oil instead of cream or butter (both of which are high in the saturated type), your body uses the healthier fat faster, your blood glucose and insulin levels stay lower, and you use more calories digesting it.

When the bad LDL cholesterol becomes oxidized, as it often does when your blood glucose levels are poorly controlled, it has the potential to damage your arteries even more. Physical activity has a greater effect on your levels of good HDL cholesterol. A high level of regular activity elevates HDL, while a sedentary state lowers it. Diabetic men who reduce their intake of refined carbohydrates have experienced improvements in both types of cholesterol, demonstrated by lower LDL and higher HDL levels.

You shouldn't avoid all types of fat, though. Two polyunsaturated fats are considered essential in your diet: omega-3 and omega-6. You will find omega-3 fats abundant in dark green, leafy vegetables (e.g., dark-colored lettuce, spinach, kale, turnip greens, etc.), canola oil, flaxseed oil, soy, some nuts (e.g. walnuts), fish, and fish oils, but only the latter two foods also contain larger amounts of two critical omega-3 fats called DHA (docosahexaenoic acid) and EPA (eicosapentanoic acid), which are critical for brain and nerve function, cardiovascular health, and more. The other essential fat, omega-6, is more abundant in the corn, sunflower, peanut, and soy oils that constitute such food products as margarine, salad dressing, and cooking oils. Although your intake of each of these omega fats can vary widely with what you eat, your health will benefit by trying to balance your intake of the two. In organically raised meat like free-range chicken and grass-fed beef, the ratio of the two essential omegas is one to one, which is recommended. In commercially raised animals, however, omega-6s are in excess, with the resulting meat often containing fourteen times more of them than omega-3s.

Fish is often touted as a heart-healthy food due to its high content of omega-3s, especially DHA and EPA. The governments of Britain and Australia are now advising healthy people to get 400 to 600 milligrams (mg) a day of DHA and EPA through consumption of fish. The American Heart Association recommends that people with heart disease supplement with 1,000 mg of DHA plus EPA because these fats lower the risk of sudden death from a heart attack; in fact, eating fish five times a week may lower your risk by 40 percent. DHA in particular may also have a beneficial effect on eye health and prevent or delay age- or diabetes-related eye diseases. Luckily, there are many delicious dishes in the Latino cuisine that use fish and other seafood. (Look for hundreds of diabetes-savvy fish recipes online at www.dlife.com/dLife/diabetic-recipes.html.)

Americans are advised to eat fatty fish like salmon, tuna, and halibut at least twice weekly, and vegetarians can supplement with DHA in algal oil (from algae). But farm-raised fish—which are becoming more prevalent in order to counteract overfishing and meet the world's growing demand for fish—contain more omega-6s than the wild type. Taking in too many omega-6s (relative to omega-3s) can actually be pro-inflammatory and may contribute to oxidative damage and the development of clogged arteries and heart disease. If you are intent on ingesting more of the healthiest omega-3s through enriched foods, take care to read food labels carefully as most manufacturers add ALA (alpha linolenic acid) from flaxseed and other sources to boost the total content. ALA is not considered as heart-healthy as DHA and EPA.

What fats should you eat?

Still confused about the recommended intake of fat in your diet? As mentioned, cutting out all fat is not likely to solve your insulin resistance or keep you from developing cardiovascular problems, and diets high in the monounsaturated type may actually improve your insulin action. Unnaturally low-fat diets can cause your liver to produce more LDL cholesterol, especially if you replace the fat calories you've removed from your diet with refined carbohydrates. The best advice is to simply cut down on your intake of saturated and trans fats by eating more foods in their natural state, such as high-fiber fruits, vegetables, legumes, and fish. If you eat a diet that is moderate in fat (30 percent of your daily calories) and saturated fat (no more than 10 percent) and avoid lower-fat versions of snack foods that have added sugar and more refined carbohydrates in them, your cholesterol levels will still go down.

What about the fat in dairy products and nuts? Some of what these contain is saturated fat, but not all of it. If you consume cheese and milk, pick lower-fat varieties because they contain fewer calories and the fat you're cutting out is mostly the saturated type. Also, keep in mind that diets rich in monounsaturated fats coming from olive oil, canola oil, and nuts are heart-healthy and do not necessarily promote weight gain. Studies have shown that if you're following a weight loss diet and eat a handful of almonds daily, you'll likely lose more weight than if you eat the same number of calories without the nuts. (Watch the sodium content, though.)

Healthy fats such as those found in fish, nuts, and olive oil don't increase levels of insulin resistance as other fats can. You can prepare delicious Latino dishes using healthy fats and oils. However, avoid eating the unhealthier fats that are found in processed foods and may be disguised as palm, coconut, or palm-kernel oil; mono- and diglycerides; stearate; palmitate; lard; vegetable shortening; and hydrogenated or partially hydrogenated oils. Oils that are more damaging to your coronary arteries and glycemic control are the ones that are usually solid or semisolid at room temperature, such as saturated fats found in meat, dairy fat, tropical oils, and trans fats manufactured by hydrogenating or partially hydrogenating liquid oils to alter their texture. You can find some brands of margarine nowadays that have been made without trans fats and enhanced with omega-3s (e.g., flaxseed oil containing ALA) that are healthier alternatives. The next fat that people are going to have to watch out for is one called inter-esterified fat, which is also manufactured and added to processed foods in place of trans fats. Preliminary studies show that this new type of altered fat is also heart-unhealthy, probably as much so as trans fats.

Although less unhealthy than once believed, your cholesterol intake should decrease as you eliminate the saturated and trans fats in your diet. Your body does use a certain amount of cholesterol, which is a waxy, fat-like substance important in cell and hormone composition, and your liver will simply make it if you don't eat enough. Cholesterol is found in all animal products, including meat, poultry, shellfish, fish, eggs, and dairy, but not in plant sources (grains, vegetables, fruits, nuts, and legumes). The cholesterol found in eggs is no longer as maligned as it once was, but since eggs contain almost 300 mg per egg yolk, it's easy to go overboard if you eat more than one yolk at a time. It is still recommended that you limit your daily cholesterol intake to no more than 300 mg per day, or no more than 100 mg per 1,000 calories. You can cook with egg whites only or use an egg substitute to lower your cholesterol intake.

Using the glycemic index (GI) when choosing carbohydrates

If you fear having to give up the carbohydrate-heavy foods you love—be it rice, beans, or something else—you may not need to worry. Many of these foods can be included as part of your diabetes meal plan. Although carbohydrates raise your blood glucose levels, you just need to learn how to choose them wisely and "budget" your intake.

We mentioned previously that how rapidly a carbohydrate is digested affects your body's insulin responses and ability to control your blood sugar. This concept is known as the glycemic index (GI). The more rapidly a food is broken down, the sooner the carbohydrate is turned into glucose and released into your bloodstream. To deal with the influx of glucose coming from carbohydrates with higher GI values, your pancreas must release a large amount of insulin to remove that excess blood glucose. If you have diabetes or prediabetes, your body may not be able to respond to these glucose spikes with enough insulin.

GI values are usually scaled from 0 to 100, with glucose (the simple sugar that all carbohydrate breaks down into in your body) being the most rapidly absorbed (a GI of 100). If a food has a high GI value, then your blood glucose will rise rapidly after eating it; a lower GI value means that the food causes less of an increase in blood sugar. High-GI foods have a GI value of seventy or above, and most contain highly refined flour or added sugars; some examples are breakfast cereals, pretzels, sugary candy, crackers, and bread. White potatoes may be natural, but they are also digested rapidly. Other carbs cause less of a spike in blood glucose levels and are generally easier for your body to handle, as long as you eat moderate amounts. Sweet potatoes, rice (white or brown), oatmeal, and white sugar have GI values in the range of fifty-six to sixty-nine, which makes them medium-GI foods. Most whole fruits, fructose (fruit sugar), dairy products, legumes (beans), and pasta (white or whole wheat) fall into the low-GI category (55 and lower). You will find a list of common foods, their GI values, and total carbohydrate loads in Appendix B; alternately, the latest GI database is accessible through www.glycemicindex.com (you have

to search each food separately) or found in its entirety at www
.mendosa.com/gilists.htm.

When considering GI, remember that the GI of a particular
food can differ from one person to the next, and it can also be affected by the type and amount of carbohydrate, fat, and protein a
food contains; the amount of fiber and the nature of any starches in
it; its preparation (raw or cooked); its ripeness; and its acidity. For
instance, the glycemic response to diced potatoes is somewhat
lower than to mashed potatoes, and thick linguine has a lower GI
value than thin spaghetti. Cooking in general (and overcooking in
particular) raises the GI value of foods, so al dente pasta is always
better. Highly acidic foods (e.g., vinegar) can lower the GI value of
another food when consumed in combination. Another good example of how a food's preparation affects its GI value is potato
salad. If it's made the day before, tossed with vinaigrette dressing,
and kept cold overnight, it will have a much lower GI than potatoes freshly cooked and served steaming hot. Cold storage increases the resistant starch content (carbohydrates that are hard to
digest) by more than a third, and the acid in lemon juice, lime juice,
or vinegar will slow stomach emptying.

As you can see, there are many factors to consider. We do know,
however, that an excessive intake of high-GI carbohydrate foods
can increase insulin resistance even in people without diabetes.
The GI values of foods have mainly been determined in nondiabetic individuals, so their effect may be exaggerated if your body
releases less insulin or your insulin action is impaired. If anything,
GI tables more than likely underestimate rather than overestimate
the glycemic spikes caused by most carbohydrate-rich foods if you
have diabetes.

Research also supports the benefits of lowering the glycemic effect of your meals. For example, in overweight adults, insulin re-

sistance can be decreased when they consume a low-GI, whole-grain diet compared to a refined, "white" diet. Moreover, a 2004 study of type 2 diabetic men following a low-GI diet (<40 on the GI scale) demonstrated an improvement in their blood glucose control, enhanced insulin action, and lower blood fats after only four weeks. Such positive results overwhelmingly support the argument that the GI is an appropriate guide to eating more nutritious foods whether you have diabetes, prediabetes, or insulin resistance, or if you just want to stay healthy.

Factoring in glycemic load (GL)

You can still eat some carbohydrates, just not gargantuan portions. When it comes to carbs, portion size does matter. Glycemic load (GL) is a measure of both GI value and total carbohydrate intake in a typical serving. A GL of twenty or more is high, eleven to nineteen is medium, and ten or less is low. Foods that have a low GL almost always have a lower GI value, with some exceptions: Watermelon has a high GI value (72), but the carbohydrate content per serving of this fruit is minimal, making its glycemic load (4) low. You have to watch how big a slice of watermelon you eat, however, because a serving is just over a cup (8 ounces). Popcorn also has a higher GI value (72), but it takes a lot of popcorn to equal a 50 gram serving, which has a GL of just 8.

Eating a high-GL diet for many years substantially increases your risk for developing diabetes, particularly if you are overloading on refined carbohydrates. Paying attention to your GL is even more important if you have diabetes. Then you want to keep your blood sugar lower because a high-GI/GL diet will most likely worsen your insulin resistance and overtax your body's ability to supply enough insulin. Try to limit your intake of foods with both a high or medium GI value and a high GL. Any carbohydrate-heavy meal with a high GL will require more insulin, but if the GI value is not also high—as is generally the case with high-fiber foods—your blood sugar will stay lower. In Latino cooking, an example of a higher GL, lower GI meal is one centered around legumes, which are rich in protein and fiber, as well as carbohydrate with a lower glycemic effect. Another benefit of limiting your total carbohydrate intake is that a low-GL, high-fiber diet raises circulating levels of adiponectin, an anti-inflammatory hormone released by fat cells that can increase your insulin action and improve your blood glucose control. A low GI/GL diet plan results in weight loss as well.

The main take-home messages regarding glycemic index and glycemic load includes the following: (1) choose slowly absorbed carbohydrates, not necessarily just a smaller amount of total carbs; (2) use the GI to identify your best carbohydrate choices, choosing lower GI ones; and (3) limit your portion size when eating carb-rich foods like rice, pasta, beans, or noodles to limit the overall GL of your diet. It is almost impossible to avoid spikes in your blood sugar levels if you eat a large quantity of carbohydrate at any one time, even if you're just eating legumes or pasta, both with a lower GI.

Many diabetic individuals who have to cover their food intake with insulin count carbs, meaning that they try to estimate the actual amount of carbohydrates in grams (Table 3.1) that they are eating and give themselves specific doses of insulin to cover it based on an insulin-to-carbohydrate ratio that works for them. For people who have diabetes, even sugar-free desserts can have a major effect on their blood sugar due to their high content of refined carbohydrates. Thus you must take every kind of carbohydrate into account if you plan on controlling your blood sugar.

Table 3.1: Portion Size, Calories, and Carbohydrate Content of Some
Common Foods

	Portion Size	Calories	Carbohydrates (grams)
Apple	1 small	60	15
Avocado	2 ounces	45	0
Banana	1/2 medium	60	15
Beans (legumes, most varieties)	1/2 cup	80	15
Bread, white or wheat	1 slice	80	15
Broccoli	1/2 cup cooked, 1 cup raw	25	5
Carrots	1/2 cup cooked, 1 cup raw	25	5
Cauliflower	1/2 cup cooked, 1 cup raw	25	5
Cheese (most types)	1 ounce	105	0
Cherries	12	60	15
Chicken, white meat (no skin)	3 ounces	105	0
Corn	1/2 cup	80	15
Eggs	1	75	0
Enchilada, meat	1	213	21
Fish, baked or grilled (most types)	3 ounces	90	0
Grapefruit	1/2 medium	60	15
Grapes	15 medium	60	15
Lettuce (all types)	1 cup	25	5
Margarine	1 tablespoon	100	0
Meat (most types)	3 ounces	165	0
Melon	1 cup	60	15
Milk, soy or skim	1 cup	90	12
Milk, 1%	1 cup	105	12
Milk, 2%	1 cup	120	12
Milk, whole	1 cup	150	12
Nuts (most types)	1 ounce	170	3–8
Olives, black	8 large	45	0
Orange	1 medium	60	15

(continues)

Table 3.1 *(continued)*

	Portion Size	Calories	Carbohydrates (grams)
Pasta, cooked	1/3 cup	80	15
Peanut butter	1 tablespoon	94	3
Pineapple	3/4 cup	60	15
Potato, sweet	1/2 cup	80	15
Potato, white	1/2 medium	80	15
Raspberries	1 cup	60	15
Rice, cooked	1/3 cup	80	15
Sausage	3 ounces	330	2
Seafood (most types)	3 ounces	85	0
Spinach	1/2 cup cooked, 1 cup raw	25	5
Strawberries	1 1/4 cup	60	15
Tortilla, regular	1	80	15

Importantly, the effect of a low-GI food carries over to the next meal, reducing its glycemic impact. A breakfast eaten after a low-GI dinner the previous evening will produce less blood glucose fluctuation, as will a lunch eaten after a low-GI breakfast. This is known as the "second meal effect." Always aim to eat at least one lower-GI food that will help counterbalance the other foods in a meal. For instance, if you combine high-GI bakery products with protein foods and low-GI carbohydrates (e.g., legumes or fruit), the overall GI value of your meal will be medium. Also, if you have recently eaten foods with a high GL or high GI value, exercising to use up a significant amount of stored muscle glycogen before you eat again will help moderate the impact of your next meal. Essentially, using up carbohydrates in muscles (glycogen) through physical activity gives the next carbohydrates you eat storage space outside of your bloodstream.

LORENA DRAGO
Going beyond beans and rice with diet and diabetes education

Latina certified diabetes educator (CDE) and registered dietitian Lorena Drago does not have diabetes herself, but she has made it her mission to help people with diabetes learn to eat right and live well. For starters, Lorena wrote the book *Beyond Beans and Rice: The Caribbean Latino Guide to Eating Healthy with Diabetes*, which was published by the American Diabetes Association in 2006. To make sure everyone understands, the book is bilingual: English on one side and Spanish on the other. In addition, Lorena has created two nutritional tools for people with diabetes: a set of measuring cups that have the carbohydrate and calorie content of traditional favorite foods on the side and a set of cards with pictures of traditional Latino foods on one side and the nutritional information about them on the other. These tools can even help health educators who are not familiar with Latino foods teach their patients how to create a meal within their own carbohydrate budget.

Lorena has found that many of her diabetic patients (who primarily have type 2) struggle with food choices. She says, "I think taking medications, monitoring, and keeping appointments is very simple compared to making 'the right food choices,' especially because food is ubiquitous and tied to many Latino cultural activities. Most of my patients feel deprived when they can't eat certain foods or as much as they would like of certain foods." She finds many of them are willing to learn, though. "They ask questions, read books and magazines, and learn to modify certain dietary habits; for example, they switch to sugar-free soda if they drank regular; they use lower carbohydrate foods in place of starchy root vegetables; and they use olive oil instead of corn."

On the topic of glucose monitoring, Lorena tells her patients, "Monitoring is the GPS of diabetes. You need to know where you are so you know when you reach your destination." She confirms that monitoring works when people are "able to understand how food, medication, physical activity, and other factors impact their blood sugar levels." She finds, however, that not all patients are equally dedicated to using this tool. The frequency of their monitoring depends on their financial status, the medications they take, and their attitude.

With regard to what specific barriers the diabetic Latino community faces in managing diabetes, Lorena says, "I feel we ask most Latino patients to change too many things at the same time, and that leads to frustration. It's best to help people adjust to their new lives one step at a time." To do so, she believes, they need access to practical information about controlling diabetes, including information about the benefits of properly using medications like metformin, glitazones, sulfonylureas like glyburide, Byetta, cholesterol and blood pressure pills, and even aspirin therapy. (These medications are discussed fully in Chapter 7.)

Finally, Lorena Drago believes that diabetic individuals will do better if they practice managing their health problems. "No one expects an Olympic star to achieve greatness by only practicing the sport a few hours in one year," she comments. "However, we expect patients with diabetes to achieve positive health outcomes after two to three hours of diabetes education." Instead, she believes that they need continuous care and support. "I believe those patients who have ongoing support and are taught effective problem solving skills and relapse recovery can be very successful in managing their diabetes."

Living la vida buena *without sugar?*

You may have noticed in the GI/GL table that white sugar has only a medium-GI value and a low GL. While eating too much sugar is not a direct cause of diabetes, the effects of white sugar and other refined carbohydrates are not trivial. As you have learned, refined carbohydrates are a source of empty calories that contain few essential nutrients and lots of calories, making higher-GI carbohydrates certain to throw off your blood glucose balance. It's not necessary to give up white and other refined sugars completely, but it would greatly behoove you to strictly limit your intake of them.

One of the easiest ways to start lowering the sugar content of your diet and improving its glycemic effect is to reduce or eliminate your intake of all regular soft drinks, juice, fruit juice drinks, and sugar-sweetened iced tea or lemonade. By simply not drinking calorie-filled sodas, you're likely to consume 10 percent fewer calories on a daily basis. It's infinitely better to substitute water, diet soft drinks (especially the noncaffeinated, noncola varieties), or other artificially sweetened beverages such as Crystal Light. Your blood glucose will surely suffer if you drink sugar-filled sodas or juices. Starting by cutting out some of the more obvious sources of refined sugar in your diet also helps wean you off of them, which is better than trying to go "cold turkey" with sugar consumption. The latest research suggests that sugar (and carbohydrates) may actually be addictive by causing the release of brain hormones like dopamine in response to its intake.

Cutting back on refined sugar in foods also involves being a more informed and careful consumer who identifies added sugars by reading food labels and carefully checking all food ingredients. Food and drink manufacturers must list ingredients in order of descending weight. In many products, refined sugar would come first if companies had not found so many creative ways to disguise it by adding four or five different sweeteners that then appear lower on the list of ingredients. Added sugar equivalents include sucrose, dextrose, high-fructose corn syrup, corn syrup, glucose, fructose, maltose, levulose, honey, brown sugar, and molasses.

Choosing "sugar-free" and "fat-free" varieties of foods is not necessarily better as the former are rarely sugarless (as you will discover when you read the labels looking for possible sugar equivalents), and most are far from being calorie-free or even reduced calorie. Such products are typically high in fat and not beneficial to anyone with diabetes. Along the same lines, fat-free products are usually higher in sugar. Whenever food manufacturers remove flavor enhancers such as fat or sugar, they have to replace them with something else, so if fat is taken out, sugar is usually added and vice versa.

Sugar alcohols, such as sorbitol and mannitol (and others that end in "-ol"), are absorbed slowly or poorly to some extent (thus reducing their GI value), but they still contain almost the same amount of carbohydrate or GL as plain old sugar. Sorbitol is often used in candy products like sugarless gummy snacks, and except for taking longer to metabolize, the carbohydrate effects and calorie count are similar to those of white sugar. (Incidentally, the malabsorbed part of most sugar alcohols has a laxative effect, and even 10 grams of sorbitol or mannitol can send you running for the bathroom.) Lactilol, an altered form of milk sugar found in products like Hershey's sugar-free dark chocolate candy bars, is also neither truly sugarless nor calorie-free. Its calorie content is equal to that of a regular Hershey's chocolate bar, and a similar number of carbohydrates will eventually be absorbed, albeit more slowly, into the bloodstream. A slower rate of absorption may control your diabetes better, but be careful not to overeat such foods just because you mistakenly believe that they don't contain as many grams of carbohydrates or calories.

Using artificial or low-calorie sweeteners, however, may help you reduce your calorie intake and stick to a healthier meal plan. Such sweeteners reduce your intake of high-GI carbohydrates when used in place of sugar to sweeten coffee, tea, cereal, or fruit. They add sweetness without adding calories. Approved artificial sweeteners include saccharin, aspartame, acesulfame potassium, sucralose, neotame, and tagatose, to name a few. Sucralose (marketed as Splenda) is currently the most popular and has largely replaced aspartame (NutraSweet) in many products. Some people are sensitive to NutraSweet and have negative reactions like headache or stomach upset when they consume it. If that is the case for you, try Splenda or another sugar substitute.

Strategies for Better Controlling Your Blood Sugar

- Pay careful attention to glycemic index and glycemic load when choosing foods.
- Severely limit the quantity of white foods that you consume, including bread, rice, potatoes, sugar, and pasta.
- Limit intake of any type of carbohydrate to no more than two servings at one time (e.g., 1 cup cooked pasta, 2/3 cup rice, 2 slices of bread, or 3 ounces of potatoes).
- Balance glycemic load with greater intake of fiber-rich, lower-calorie foods (like vegetables) at meals, and eat them first to fill up quicker.
- Always eat whole fruits rather than drinking fruit juices, and limit your intake of dried fruits to appropriate serving sizes.
- Limit your drinks to plain water; noncaloric flavored water; diet, phosphate-free soft drinks; and occasionally low-fat milk.
- Limit your intake of saturated and trans fats, replacing them with healthier monounsaturated fats found in olive and canola oils.
- Watch out for calorie-dense, hidden fats in margarine, butter, mayonnaise, gravy, salad dressing, sour cream, cream, whole milk products, and meat.
- Watch out for excessive added sugars in many low-fat and fat-free foods.
- Wait at least fifteen minutes before getting a second helping to allow your stomach to register its fullness with your brain, or plan a light snack for two to three hours afterward.
- Never feel obligated to finish all of the food on your plate, with the possible exception of your vegetables (if prepared without much added fat).
- Pack your own lunch and snacks for school, work, and everywhere else.
- Avoid eating at buffet-style or all-you-can-eat restaurants. If you visit one, limit yourself to one plateful of salad and vegetables, followed by a smaller plateful of entrée items.
- Allow yourself one small treat a day, but keep it moderate (no more than 150 calories).

Time to pass on coffee?

Caffeine has no calories, and it actually stimulates your metabolism somewhat, so why shouldn't you have regular coffee with breakfast, as well as diet colas, iced tea, and other caffeinated drinks throughout the day? According to the latest research, rather than improving your chances of avoiding diabetes as earlier studies had claimed, caffeine makes your body more insulin resistant. In lean, obese, and type 2 diabetic people equally, caffeine ingestion equivalent to two to three 8-ounce cups of coffee (5 mg per kilogram of body weight) per day reduces insulin sensitivity by about one-third, and the caffeine-induced decrement is still present after as many as three months of regular, moderate aerobic exercise, which usually increases insulin action.

In a 2008 study published in *Diabetes Care*, researchers presented findings about the effects of coffee on people trying to control their type 2 diabetes with diet, exercise, and oral medications only. Wearing a glucose monitor for seventy-two hours revealed that when participants drank caffeine (two cups of coffee daily), their blood sugar rose by 8 percent. Caffeine consumption also exaggerated the rise in their blood sugar after meals: by 9 percent after breakfast, 15 percent after lunch, and 26 percent after dinner. Before you load up on coffee or other caffeinated drinks, consider whether you may be able to lower your blood sugar simply by cutting such drinks out of your diet instead. Don't replace coffee with sugary drinks or lots of fruit juice, though, or your diabetes risk and blood sugar will still be elevated. Choose herbal or decaffeinated teas, decaf coffee, sugar-free hot cocoa, and low-calorie drinks instead.

How to eat more and weigh less

The best part of a high-fiber, unrefined diet is that you can eat more and weigh less. The calorie density of foods contributes most to weight gain. To lose weight, simply eat "bigger" foods, those that are bulked up by fiber and water, making them less calorie dense. Broth-based soups are generally lower in calories because of their high water and (usually) vegetable content (but watch out for sodium), and people who eat more soup often have a lower body weight for their size. Even whipped foods may fill you up better because of their additional air content. Other high-volume foods include most vegetables, whole fruits, air-popped popcorn, and lettuce-based salads (with modest amounts of salad dressing).

Here's another trick for cutting calories: If you start your meal with a salad containing three cups of lettuce and vegetables and use a low-calorie salad dressing, you will eat an average of 12 percent fewer calories at any meal. Although such small reductions may not seem like much, you end up saving 560 calories in a week, about 2,300 a month, and 29,000 in a year—equal to about eight pounds of fat!—just by adding a salad to your dinner and eating less of other foods. You eat the same volume of food but fewer calories, and you aren't left feeling hungry.

Try to avoid all-you-can-eat buffets. They're not at all helpful for people with diabetes as you'll likely eat more than you need when you're paying for an unlimited amount of food. The lack of vegetables, salad, or fresh fruit not already doctored with extra butter, oil, dressing, or other oily calories makes your blood sugar harder to control. Very large meals with high fat and carbohydrate content result in a major increase in your insulin needs. Most people with diabetes find it impossible to eat a buffet meal—even one heavy on salads and vegetables—that does not end up negatively impacting their blood sugar for many hours afterward. If you have a choice, always order off the menu, even though it may cost more, to control the size and carb content of your meal.

Another helpful practice is to graze—eat small meals and snacks throughout the day. Grazing will usually cause you to end up leaner than someone who eats less often, even if you're eating an equivalent number of calories. Eating four to six smaller meals throughout the day may keep your metabolic rate at a higher level, increasing your overall energy expenditure for each day. Eating more frequently also keeps you from getting too hungry between meals, which will make you less likely to overeat. When you eat only small amounts of food—particularly carbohydrate—at any given time, your body is more likely to be able to release enough insulin to keep your blood sugar lower.

Finally, the timing of your meals can affect your body weight and overall health, as can skipping them altogether. Breakfast serves to break your overnight fast, effectively kicking your fasting metabolism into a higher gear and lowering levels of hormones (like cortisol) that increase insulin resistance. Skipping your first meal sustains your fast and keeps your body in an energy-conserving mode, making you expend fewer calories until you eat again. In such a metabolic state, you are less responsive to insulin and your blood sugar suffers. Healthy women who eat breakfast are more insulin sensitive throughout the day than those who skip it, and breakfast abstainers also consume a larger number of calories over the course of the day in spite of not consuming breakfast calories. In fact, people who eat breakfast are usually leaner than people who skip it, and skipping breakfast increases your risk for developing type 2 diabetes.

CHAPTER 3: *En pocas palabras*

Latinos eat a variety of cuisines, reflecting their country of origin. Paying attention to the type of carbohydrates and fat that you eat can improve your health. Blood sugar levels after a meal are also affected by the glycemic effect that a food has (its glycemic index, or GI, and its glycemic load, or GL), which is largely determined by carbohydrate choices and portion sizes. Choosing healthy foods that are less refined, higher in fiber, and abundant in natural phytonutrients will improve your health and your diabetes control.

CHAPTER 4

Choosing Supplements Wisely

We hear a lot about dietary supplements and herbal remedies, much of it false or only partially true. How can you determine what is correct and what is not? You have to arm yourself with scientifically based information. When used judiciously, certain vitamins, minerals, herbs, foods, and other dietary supplements may actually help control or prevent diabetes and its complications and improve overall health. In this chapter, you will learn more about which ones you should consider—and which ones you should not.

Using herbal and folk medicine or nutritional supplements

Some Latinos believe that scares, attacks, evil eyes, spiritual works, and sorcerers can cause illnesses. Others rely on folk healers and home remedies to treat illnesses. Older Latinos often view aches and pains as part of the natural aging process. They rely on home or other remedies first, seeking out appropriate health care at a later time when it is too little, too late and simply reinforces their belief that conventional medicine is not worth pursuing. Not surprisingly, then, many Latinos turn to folk medicine and herbal remedies to cure diabetes and other health problems. While the use of folk medicine is beyond the scope of this book, in the next section we will discuss the judicious use of herbal and other over-the-counter nutritional products (including vitamins and minerals) in controlling diabetes and its complications.

Precautions about self-prescribed supplement use

Unfortunately, you can never really be certain what you are getting in the supplements you may take. Companies selling herbs are not required to demonstrate the safety or efficacy of their products, and, unlike prescription medicines, their products are not regulated by the Food and Drug Administration. Consequently, the dietary supplement industry has been outside any type of control for more than a decade despite the fact that people worldwide spend more than $60 billion a year on supplements annually.

If you decide to use home remedies or supplements, keep in mind that "herbal" or "natural" on a label does not mean that they're innocuous or harmless. In fact, many common poisons found in plants like hemlock and deadly nightshade are "natural." Some dietary supplements may have undesirable side effects, such as certain forms of ginseng that can raise blood pressure and mugwort (or mother wort) that can cause dermatitis (skin inflammation). Others can interact with prescribed medications to produce side effects or possibly negate the usual effects of the medication. For instance, people have been poisoned, in some cases fatally, by herbal preparations containing heliotropium while also taking a prescribed barbiturate. To avoid these possibilities, inform your doctor about any herbal preparations you use, especially if you take any prescribed medications for your diabetes or other health problems.

The supplements you buy may vary widely in their actual content. Some studies have even shown no ginseng in products that are sold as ginseng supplements, and the ingredients in many herbal preparations are not listed on the packaging. Even when they are, the lists may not be accurate or complete. Up to 26 percent of all dietary supplements tested in one study contained contaminants sufficient to elicit a positive drug test in competitive athletes. Others may contain harmful and even potentially fatal contaminants.

Finally, be very cautious when self-prescribing a supplement that could potentially affect your blood glucose levels. Just because a supplement is supposedly good for you, you can't assume that taking more of it is going to be better. It is possible to take in toxic amounts of substances—even natural vitamins like A and D—if you self-prescribe large doses. Again, there is no evidence as to how those supplements or herbs can interact with your current diabetes medications, so you need to be extra careful and talk with your doctor before you start taking them.

Do you need to take nutritional supplements?

We firmly believe that it's always best to obtain nutrients naturally through your foods if you can, as they contain many important compounds (e.g., flavonols, polyphenols, catechins, and lycopenes) that are not likely to be obtained in an optimal form through dietary supplements. Such supplements should neither displace a healthy amount of whole foods, such as grains, vegetables, fruits, and nuts from your diet, nor can they fully compensate for an absence of these foods. Moreover, these nutrient compounds often act in synergistic ways that can't be replicated with supplements containing only one or a few of them.

Whereas diabetes can create a special metabolic situation that may deplete certain nutrients, you may be able to compensate with healthier food choices, select nutritional supplements, and improved blood glucose control. If you are getting the recommended daily amounts of vitamins and minerals in your diet, then you may not need any supplements, which are usually only beneficial if you are truly deficient. While insulin resistance and hyperglycemia can potentially cause certain nutrient deficiencies, if you control these conditions effectively, then supplements may not be of any additional help and can be potentially harmful.

As for health claims about the benefits of specific nutritional supplements—even common recommendations to take a daily multivitamin or mineral supplement—don't believe everything you read or hear. The scientific evidence is often conflicting and inconclusive, and new studies often contradict previous ones. Recent studies reported that conjugated linoleic acid, touted as a weight-loss supplement, increases insulin resistance in obese men while other experts claimed the opposite—that it prevents insulin resistance in anyone with diabetes. We really don't know what the correct answer is yet, likewise with the need for other supplemental vitamins, minerals, and other compounds. While some experts argue that you can get everything your body needs through a nutritionally balanced diet, others assert that nutritional supplements are absolutely necessary in today's nutritionless world, especially if you have a chronic health problem like diabetes.

If you do choose to start taking a daily supplement, test its effect by having your overall blood glucose control and lipid levels tested before you start and again no sooner than three months later. If you have improvements (while keeping your diet and exercise regimens and your medications the same), the supplements may be beneficial for you. Unfortunately, if you choose to supplement with antioxidants, there is no easy way to assess their direct impact.

Certain antioxidant supplements may be beneficial

Elevated blood glucose is one of the conditions that can trigger damage caused by excess free radicals (compounds that cause oxidative damage and inflammation), and the resulting oxidative stress may contribute to any or all of the complications associated with long-term diabetes, including heart disease and eye, kidney, and nerve damage. Exercise also stimulates the production of these radicals, but it enhances your body's antioxidant enzyme systems that get rid of them. These radical compounds, if left unchecked, promote further insulin resistance and a lower insulin secretion, which is exactly what you don't want if you have diabetes or prediabetes.

Not surprisingly, antioxidant vitamins and minerals are among the most popular supplements nowadays, not just for diabetes reasons, but also to potentially slow the normal aging process. Normally, your body possesses enough antioxidant enzymes to fight most or all of the free radicals that are created. Diabetes not only increases free radical generation when your blood sugars are elevated, but it also depresses your body's natural antioxidant defenses. If your blood glucose levels are poorly controlled, you are more likely to benefit from supplemental antioxidant therapies.

Potentially, the most beneficial antioxidants for anyone with diabetes are vitamin C, vitamin E, beta-carotene, glutathione, alpha lipoic acid (LA), selenium, copper, and zinc. Diabetic complications like cataracts involve deficient glutathione levels within the lens of your eye, and nutrients like LA, vitamins E and C, and selenium can increase your levels of glutathione and its activity, allowing for better protection of your eyes and other tissues. A combination of vitamins C and E and minerals magnesium and zinc may improve the good cholesterol in people with diabetes.

Taking large supplemental doses of these nutrients can be counterproductive, though, as almost all antioxidants have been shown to have the opposite effect when you take too much. You can't overdose on antioxidants if you obtain them naturally through food, so consume them that way whenever possible. Some surprising foods and drinks contain large amounts of various antioxidants. A typical cup of hot cocoa (containing two tablespoons of pure cocoa powder) has twice as many of these health-promoting compounds (flavonoids in particular) as red wine, two to three times more than green tea, and almost five times more than black tea. Drinking cocoa hot also apparently releases more antioxidant power (but use the sugar-free variety for better diabetes control).

Is more vitamin A or beta-carotene necessary?

Beta-carotene, one compound in a family of carotenoids, can boost the activity of your tumor-scavenging, natural killer (NK) cells, which are an integral part of your cell-based immune system. Beta-carotene also helps inhibit cholesterol synthesis, facilitate cellular interactions, and stimulate enzymes to repair damaged DNA. To be active, it must be converted by your body into the active form of vitamin A (retinol), which helps maintain the health of your eyes, immune system, skin, epithelial cells (which line the organs and are where cancers start), and memory.

Taking supplements of beta-carotene is generally less effective than getting it in orange-yellow plant foods like carrots and sweet potatoes, which also contain other carotenoid compounds (e.g., alpha-carotene) that may be even more effective cancer fighters than the beta form. Recent studies suggest that synergies between carotenoids (both those that can be converted into vitamin A and those that cannot) can lower the risk of developing diabetic retinopathy, particularly if you increase your intake of lutein- and lycopene-rich fruits and vegetables (e.g., tomatoes, spinach, kale). Insulin resistance is also lower in people with higher levels of antioxidant carotenoids in their bloodstream, even when they don't have diabetes.

Megadoses of beta-carotene are generally harmless, but a balanced, healthy diet supplies more than adequate amounts. Conversely, vitamin A is toxic if you take it in large doses as a dietary supplement. Retinol is found mainly in foods such as liver, butter, cheese, egg yolks, fish liver oils, and fortified milk (Table 4.1); in fact, a single serving of liver provides 1,000 percent of the recommended daily intake. The upper limit for intake of vitamin A is 10,000 international units (IU), but beta-carotene has no limit. Focus on increasing your beta-carotene intake, which can be accomplished by eating yellow-orange vegetables and fruits, among other foods. A medium-size carrot supplies about 200 percent of the recommended daily intake.

B vitamins play many roles in your health

There are many vitamins in the B family, including thiamin (B1), riboflavin (B2), B6, niacin, B12, folate, biotin, and pantothenic acid. Considered together, the B vitamins are heavily involved in the digestion and metabolism of food, so it's not surprising that a deficiency in any of them can adversely affect your use of carbohydrates, protein, fat, and more.

Researchers have found that people with diabetes are more likely to be deficient in thiamin and that supplementation with this

Table 4.1: Dietary Sources of Essential Vitamins

Vitamin	Major Functions	Food Sources
Vitamin A	Maintains skin and mucous membranes; forms visual purple for night vision; promotes bone development; optimizes immune function; active form, retinol, often used as topical acne and wrinkle treatment	As vitamin A: meat, liver, fortified dairy products, egg yolks As beta-carotene: yellow-orange vegetables like carrots, pumpkin, squash; dark green, leafy vegetables (DGLV) like spinach, kale, and darker lettuce; tomatoes; fruits
Vitamin D	Acts as a hormone to increase calcium absorption in small intestine; promotes bone and tooth formation; active hormone, calcitriol, may also play a role in skin health, cancer and diabetes prevention, and more	Fortified dairy products, nuts and seeds, vegetable oils Note: 90 percent of vitamin D in our bodies usually comes from exposure to UV rays in sunlight
Vitamin E	Serves as an antioxidant in cell membranes to prevent damage; may help prevent certain diabetic complications like eye diseases	Vegetable oils, seeds like sunflower, nuts (e.g., almonds, peanuts, and cashews), DGLV, margarine, tomato products, sweet potatoes, wheat germ, spinach, green peas
Thiamine (B1)	Plays a central role in the metabolism of glucose; essential for normal functioning of the nervous system; depleted by excessive intake of alcohol; often low in the blood of people with diabetes	Whole grains, legumes, sunflower seeds, ham, pork, liver, enriched pastas
Riboflavin (B2)	Involved in energy production from carbohydrates and fats inside cells; helps maintain healthy skin	Liver, pork, milk, yogurt, spinach, enriched cereals, mushrooms, cottage cheese
Niacin	Important in use of stored carbohydrate in muscle cells; helps synthesize fat and block the release of free fatty acids; needed for healthy skin	Meat, poultry, fish, potatoes, enriched cereals

Vitamin	Major Functions	Food Sources
Pyridoxine (B6)	Plays central role in protein, fat, and carbohydrate metabolism; necessary for formation of hemoglobin and red blood cells to carry oxygen	Widely distributed in all types of foods, including liver, chicken, potatoes, sweet potatoes, bananas, fruit, DGLV
Biotin	Involved in the metabolism of carbohydrates, protein, and fat; aids in formation of glucose	Liver, egg yolks, legumes (e.g., peas, beans), DGLV
Folate	Critical role in formation of DNA; essential for formation of red blood cells; helps prevent neural tube defects in fetus early in pregnancy	DGLV, asparagus, avocados, whole grains, legumes, beets
Pantothenic acid	Plays a central role in energy metabolism; important for the synthesis of a neurotransmitter for muscles	Widely distributed in natural plant and animal products, especially in organ meats, eggs, legumes, yeast, whole grains
Vitamin B12	Essential for synthesis of DNA in cells; works with folate to form red blood cells; essential for formation of protective myelin sheath around nerve cells; involved in metabolism of homocysteine	Meat, poultry, fish, dairy products Note: B12 is not found in any plant sources
Vitamin C	Serves as an strong antioxidant; has role in formation of collagen (in connective tissues); involved in formation of adrenaline and other stress hormones; increases iron absorption from food and helps with red blood cell formation; needed for wound healing and scar tissue formation	Citrus fruits, bell peppers, peaches, strawberries, DGLV
Vitamin K	Forms compounds essential for blood clotting to prevent hemorrhaging; helps strengthen bones as well	DGLV, cauliflower, cabbage, soybeans, canola oil Note: The majority of vitamin K comes from friendly bacteria in the intestines

vitamin may prevent a number of diabetic complications and improve insulin action in people with type 2 diabetes. Niacin is used in therapeutic doses to help lower cholesterol levels, and low blood levels of vitamin B12 are linked to lower bone density in the spines of women and the hips of men. Low intake of folate has been associated with an increased risk of fetal defects (related to neural tube development) in pregnant women, as well as a higher risk for thinning bones and heart disease in older individuals, although taking too much of it may not be good either as large doses of folate can mask a deficiency of vitamin B12 and cause other symptoms like nausea. Biotin deficiencies have not been documented, but people with diabetes often have lower levels than their nondiabetic counterparts. Moreover, vitamin B6 and others in the B family may be effective in preventing the formation of advanced glycation end products, which are associated with high blood sugar and diabetic complications.

Make sure that your daily diet contains at least 100 percent of all of the B vitamins, and consider taking a general B supplement if you believe your diet to be lacking in any of them. Supplemental doses are generally harmless as most excess B vitamins are lost in the urine, but taking megadoses of them is neither necessary nor advised. In addition, talk to your doctor about potentially supplementing with thiamin and benfotiamine, a derivative of vitamin B1 (thiamin) with additional antioxidant properties, as it has been used therapeutically to treat neuropathic pain along with preventing other complications, improving insulin action, and lowering cholesterol levels. In some individuals with diabetes, supplementing with a combination of biotin (2 mg) and chromium picolinate (600 micrograms, or mcg) has been shown to reduce bad cholesterol and improve blood glucose control.

What vitamin C may do for your antioxidant status

Ascorbic acid, otherwise known as vitamin C, is a water-soluble vitamin with strong antioxidant qualities. Consider how the exposed surfaces of a sliced apple start to turn brown when exposed to the oxygen in the air, but if you coat the apple slices with lemon or orange juice, both of which are high in vitamin C, they stay the same color. This simple example shows how powerful an antioxidant this vitamin is. While true deficiencies of this vitamin are rare in the United States, lower blood levels of vitamin C have been found in those who are insulin resistant and at high risk for developing type 2 diabetes, and at least one study has suggested that daily supplements (250 to 500 mg) may prevent or at least reduce peripheral neuropathy (nerve damage in feet and hands) in people with diabetes.

Although this vitamin is generally considered to be less effective in combating diabetic complications than vitamin E or other antioxidants, if you use it as a supplement, it will likely help reduce your blood pressure, improve the elasticity of your arterial walls, and reduce your risk of heart disease. It also helps prevent and treat diabetic eye diseases, including cataracts and glaucoma (the second leading cause of new blindness), likely because oxidative stress is a major factor in the development of these health problems. You can easily take in the recommended dose of 200 mg per day through fruits and vegetables naturally and in processed foods as a preservative (ascorbate or ascorbic acid). Taking megadoses of vitamin C is not recommended, though, as 1,000 mg per day or more may contribute to the formation of kidney stones, result in rebound scurvy (ironically, a disease that normal doses of vitamin C typically prevent) when you stop taking it, and possibly worsen blood glucose levels.

Vitamin D, the sunshine vitamin

Recently vitamin D has been recognized as a critical hormone that has many functions, and experts have suggested that as much as 50 percent of the world's population may be at risk of a deficiency. We have long known that it increases absorption of dietary calcium to promote bone health and muscle strength, along with adequate intake of vitamin K, calcium, magnesium, and zinc. Deficient levels of vitamin D likely have a much greater negative impact on people with diabetes than was originally suspected, though, contributing to impairments in insulin secretion and action—particularly during the winter months when your vitamin D levels may be low. The active form of vitamin D, calcitriol, affects the health of your immune system, and a deficiency may contribute to the development of autoimmune-based type 1 diabetes, which is much less common in the countries closest to the equator where exposure to sunlight is greater. New evidence suggests that low vitamin D status is even a risk factor for type 2 diabetes and prediabetes because a deficiency may worsen pancreatic beta cell function.

Most foods do not naturally contain any of this vitamin, making it difficult to get enough of it in your diet. It can be obtained through fortified dairy products, margarine, and fish oils. One glass of vitamin D–fortified milk or soy milk will provide 25 percent of the recommended daily intake. However, the most effective way to have enough active vitamin D is through exposure to sunlight, as UV-B rays convert vitamin D3 into its active form. For this to happen, you must expose at least your hands, arms, and face to sunlight two to three times per week (without sunscreen on). Those with lighter skin can likely get the UV exposure they need in about ten to fifteen minutes during the warmer months of the year, but darker-skinned people have to spend up to a couple of hours in the sun to make enough vitamin D. Longer exposure is also needed during the winter; therefore, your vitamin D may be deficient during the winter months, especially if you live in northern latitudes where UV-B rays are not sufficient for many months during the year. Getting older also negatively impacts your skin's ability to produce the active form of vitamin D when exposed to sunshine.

If you're concerned about being outside without using sunscreen, keep in mind that the risk of getting skin cancer is low from the recommended level of sun exposure, which is minimal, and that higher vitamin D levels actually protect you against the development of skin melanomas. If you block too much of the sun's rays (or stay inside too much), you may actually be increasing your risk of skin (and other, deadlier) cancer rather than preventing it, or diabetes for that matter. Few older adults actually reach the recommended daily levels of vitamin D intake. For this reason, the National Academy of Sciences has set the latest vitamin D daily intake recommendations on an age-related scale: 200 IU (the amount found in two 8-ounce glasses of milk) for those nineteen to fifty years of age; 400 IU for those fifty-one to seventy; and 600 IU for people seventy and older. Many scientists now believe that your intake should be at least 1,000 IU or higher, regardless of your age. At this time, the tolerable upper intake is 2,000 IU for all adults, although toxic levels are caused by 10,000 IU or higher per day.

The potential benefits of vitamin E

One of the four essential fat-soluble vitamins, vitamin E is composed of a group of eight tocopherols, or compounds that are potent antioxidants. Due to its effects on cell membranes, this vitamin can prevent the oxidation of good fats found in various membranes in red blood cells, nerves, and lungs; reduce plaque formation in arteries; and reduce your risk of diabetes complications, including the more common ones associated with eyes (cataract formation), nerves (tingling, numbness, and pain), muscles (weakness and atrophy), and immune cells (infections). Low levels of vitamin E in the blood have also been associated with a greater risk of developing type 2 diabetes.

If you're trying to take in more vitamin E naturally through foods, keep in mind that cooking and food processing may destroy it, making it difficult for you to consume adequate amounts. Supplements may not be the answer either, though. Research has suggested that taking vitamin E as a supplement may be ineffective for preventing cardiovascular disease and, in some cases, may contribute to the development of heart failure. Moreover, combining its intake with Lipitor (a cholesterol-lowering drug) may have detrimental effects. Vitamin E supplements, most of which contain only the alpha tocopherol form, are less effective than getting all of the tocopherol compounds (alpha, delta, gamma, and others) at once like you do in foods. A few more expensive supplements contain at least several forms of these tocopherols, but they may or may not be worth the extra money. You can take up to 800 IU or mg safely as a daily supplement. If you are taking Coumadin (a blood thinner) or aspirin, check with your doctor about whether supplementing with this vitamin is advised.

What about the antioxidant power of glutathione and alpha lipoic acid?

Glutathione is the main antioxidant enzyme found in all of your cells, and, along with alpha lipoic acid (LA), is the most important antioxidant in your body. Glutathione protects the DNA in your cell nuclei from being oxidized. Diabetes can increase your body's requirements for both glutathione and LA, and although your body can synthesize both from amino acids (protein building blocks) found abundantly in foods like asparagus, avocados, spinach, strawberries, peaches, melons, and citrus fruits, it may not always make enough to meet your needs. LA increases glutathione levels by helping cells absorb a critical amino acid needed for its synthesis, and it works to prevent stroke, heart attacks, peripheral nerve damage, and cataracts, as well as memory loss, cancer, and aging effects. Spinach (raw or cooked) is the best source of this nutrient, also found naturally in small amounts in broccoli, tomatoes, potatoes, peas, and Brussels sprouts. Spinach is especially touted for its ability to fight diabetic cataracts and macular degeneration (the leading cause of blindness in all adults).

Diabetes likely increases your need for these natural antioxidants by depleting glutathione levels when your blood sugars are elevated, which can lead to diabetic cataracts and other health problems. LA supplements may normalize diabetes-induced kidney dysfunction and damage to nerve cells, where it additionally promotes nerve fiber regeneration and stimulates a substance known as nerve growth factor. Other researchers found LA to inhibit the formation of lesions in arteries, lower levels of fat (triglycerides) in blood, reduce inflammation in blood vessels, and reduce weight gain—in mice, at least. In Germany, it has been used for years to treat painful diabetic neuropathy in the feet and hands, and it can also improve autonomic (central) neuropathy. Most people can safely take 600 mg once or twice daily for relief of symptoms.

Do you need extra chromium?

Chromium helps insulin bind to receptors in fat and muscle and enhances your total number of insulin receptors and their activity. If your blood glucose levels are normal, extra intake of chromium has minimal effect. But if you are continually hyperglycemic, this mineral

MARIANA GÓMEZ HOYOS
Living with type 1 diabetes and helping to empower others with diabetes through the Mexico Diabetes Federation

Mexico resident Mariana Gómez Hoyos has been living for most of her twenty-eight years with type 1 diabetes—since the tender age of six—and she tries to help educate others with diabetes through her work with the Mexico Diabetes Federation. She emphasizes the importance of recognizing the early symptoms of diabetes because she herself was not diagnosed quickly enough and ended up in a life-threatening coma for a week as a result. "I remember having gone through all the symptoms (of diabetes) described in books for more than three months, but the pediatrician did not know about diabetes and was unable to relate them to diabetes," she recalls. "The coma I experienced due to diabetic ketoacidosis could have been avoided if the pediatrician had been aware of basic diabetic symptoms and signs."

Nowadays, she tries to follow a diet with a moderate carbohydrate intake—usually no more than 60 grams per day and 1,100 calories. She's also interested in learning more about the potential health benefits of a lower-carb diet for people with diabetes. "I have to read more and study this possibility with my diabetes expert team," she says. "I have to analyze the pros and cons soon." To cover her food intake, she uses a rapid-acting insulin analog delivered with an insulin pump, and she also takes Galvus for insulin resistance.

Mariana recognizes the challenges that she and other Latinos face in caring for their diabetes. "Diabetes is a 24/7 job," she remarks, "and I definitely can say that I work for my diabetes. Sometimes our salary is just not enough to pay for the treatments that we need. Insulin is expensive; glycemic control is as well." She gives her own main barriers as time and cost. She sometimes feels that she needs more time to devote to managing her diabetes, which involves testing her blood glucose at least twelve times a day, exercising, finding the correct food choices, and more. She says, "I need time to get enough money to take care of my diabetes. And sometimes if I work too much, I won't have time to get my diabetes in order."

About her home country of Mexico she remarks, "Diabetes is still in the shadows in our country. Doctors and other specialists do not recognize diabetes the way that they should. We [at the Mexico Diabetes Federation] have to grant scholarships, courses, and other educational materials to get them more familiar with it." She acknowledges that medical treatments for diabetes in Mexico's public clinics are not appropriate because the clinics don't always offer insulin, glucose testing supplies, or other things that may be expensive but necessary to prevent diabetic complications. Admittedly, lifestyle choices are contributing to the growing number of people in her country with this disease, but, as she remarks, "We need to make the government understand the importance of changing our lifestyles for the better in our country. We have to work on our health systems, train, teach, and learn more about diabetes."

Teaching others about diabetes has become her passion because of the number of times she has had to seek out information and care on her own over the years. Mariana remembers visiting a doctor when she first got pregnant, and his only comment to her was, "You shouldn't be pregnant. Diabetic patients should not have permission to have babies. You'll certainly have complications, and so will your baby." He didn't even ask her if she took good care of her diabetes. Today, she is blessed with a healthy two-year-old son. As she says, "Diabetes is not an obstacle, although I had to be obsessive with treating my diabetes to stay in good health during my pregnancy. Most of us will have a healthy future after all." All it takes for good diabetes control is access to information and tools.

may help reduce your blood glucose levels by improving your insulin action. Taken alone or with zinc, it may also improve your body's antioxidant capacity and cholesterol levels.

Low chromium levels are associated with a greater risk of heart attack, and supplements may reduce your risk of fatal heart arrhythmias. Although a severe deficiency of this mineral is rare, studies have shown lower blood levels in people with diabetes.

Chromium can be obtained through foods naturally (Table 4.2), but if you take a supplement, doses of less than 1,000 mcg daily appear safe for short-term use. Just to be on the safe side, don't exceed 200 mcg per day if you are going to supplement for a long time. As mentioned previously, taken in combination with biotin (one of the B vitamins), 600 mcg of this mineral may also help lower cholesterol and glucose levels, particularly if your diabetes is not well controlled. High doses of chromium picolinate can result in toxicity, but newer forms of synthetic chromium that are less toxic are being investigated.

Magnesium helps your metabolism run better

Magnesium, the fourth most abundant mineral in the body, is involved in over three hundred metabolic reactions in the body, including energy production, synthesis of genetic materials (DNA and RNA), protein production, and bone health. It helps control blood pressure, regulates the rhythm of your heart, prevents muscle cramps, and improves the action of your insulin. A magnesium deficiency can interfere with your binding of insulin, uptake of glucose into cells, and glucose use, resulting in a decrease of your body's insulin action and a higher risk for developing type 2 diabetes (if you don't have it already). In people with diabetes, low magnesium levels have been linked to a higher incidence of retinopathy and depression, as well as poorer blood sugar control.

This mineral is widely distributed in foods, including unprocessed grains, nuts, dark chocolate, and legumes. If your diabetes control is currently less than optimal, you may want to consider taking a daily magnesium supplement, along with eating a healthy diet. Like zinc, it can be depleted through excessive urination resulting from poorly controlled diabetes or excessive sweating (such as during exercise), and if you are getting frequent muscle cramps, you may be deficient. Taking too much magnesium can cause transient diarrhea, but is otherwise safe. If you have kidney failure, though, you will need to restrict your intake. Don't take more than 350 mg daily, and if your diabetes is well controlled, you may not need to supplement.

Selenium in foods is better than in supplements

This trace mineral is essential for the proper functioning of numerous enzymes in your body, particularly an antioxidant enzyme called glutathione peroxidase, which works along with vitamin E to prevent damage to the membranes of your red blood cells (among other membranes). Selenium may help prevent diabetic cataracts, heart disease (by preventing oxidation of LDL cholesterol), and prostate, colon, and lung cancers. The recommended daily intake of selenium is currently 55 mcg, which you can obtain through foods. If you take it as a supplement, your dose should not exceed 200 mcg daily, or it may impair the synthesis of thyroid hormones that elevate your metabolism. A recent study in mice also found that having higher levels of selenium may be associated with the onset of type 2 diabetes, so don't supplement with this mineral unless you are truly deficient.

Vanadium's potential effects on your azúcar sanguinea

The trace mineral vanadium may be able to lower your blood glucose levels by decreasing your liver's production of glucose while improving your insulin action, making it a potentially effective—although still unproven—treatment for diabetes. Treatment with vanadyl sulfate has also been shown to increase glutathione levels in the kidneys of diabetic rats. It has not been found to be deficient in humans,

Table 4.2: Dietary Sources of Essential Minerals

Mineral	Major Functions	Food Sources
Calcium	Involved in bone formation, enzyme activation, muscle contraction, nerve transmission, and heart function	Dairy products, dark green, leafy vegetables (DGLV), tofu, soy products, small fish with bones (e.g., sardines)
Iron	Main component of hemoglobin in red blood cells that carries oxygen in blood; important in oxidative metabolism	Ferrous form (better absorbed): meat, poultry, fish, seafood; Ferric form: DGLV, legumes, raisins, enriched cereals
Magnesium	Component of over 300 enzymes; important in protein synthesis; plays central role in glucose metabolism; involved in smooth muscle contraction and high blood pressure; often deficient in people with diabetes	Widely distributed in foods, but highest in seafood, nuts, DGLV, bananas, whole grains, semisweet chocolate, legumes
Chromium	Enhances insulin action in the body and potentiates use of glucose; involved in fat and protein metabolism as well; may affect cholesterol metabolism	Meat, organ meats, shellfish (e.g., oysters), cheese, whole grains, bran cereals, asparagus, green beans, broccoli, beer
Potassium	Works with sodium and chloride to maintain body fluid balance; helps transport glucose into the muscles for use or storage; critical for nerve impulse transmission and muscle contraction	Fresh, whole foods like bananas, potatoes, melons, avocados, salmon, lima beans
Selenium	Part of an antioxidant enzyme system to prevent cellular and oxidative damage in the body; often works with vitamin E	Brazil nuts, seafood, organ meats, grains grown in selenium-rich soil (found in most of the United States)
Zinc	Involved with over 300 enzymes to facilitate energy metabolism; important in protein synthesis, immune function, sexual maturation, bone formation, and certain senses (taste and smell)	Oysters and other shellfish, meats, poultry, whole grains, dairy products, semisweet chocolate, nuts and seeds

Mineral	Major Functions	Food Sources
Copper	Allows for proper use of iron and hemoglobin; involved in formation of connective tissues in body; part of an antioxidant enzyme system; involved in oxidative energy production	Beef, shellfish, whole grains, baking chocolate, mushrooms, nuts and seeds, legumes, potatoes, avocados, broccoli, bananas
Limit Intake:		
Sodium	Helps maintain body fluid balance; . causes body water retention; critical for nerve impulse transmission and muscle contraction	All processed foods, soups, canned vegetables, lunch meat, pickles, salty snacks
Phosphorus	Important component of bones; plays role in acid-base balance in blood; helps activate B vitamins; found in all cells; too much in diet can cause calcium bone losses	Colas (containing phosphoric acid)

though, and there is no recommended daily intake. The best way to receive enough of this trace mineral is through your food intake. Good food sources of vanadium include shellfish, whole-grain products, parsley, mushrooms, and black pepper. The average American diet supplies 15 to 30 mcg of vanadium daily, but remember that it is not considered essential. If you take supplements in larger doses, you may end up with diarrhea and toxicity, making it better to get enough through your natural food sources.

Zinc may affect insulin release

The mineral zinc is a component of more than three hundred enzymes, many of which are involved in glucose metabolism. A mild dietary zinc deficiency is thought to be common in the United States, particularly if your intake of its sources—animal proteins found in oysters and other shellfish, meats, and poultry—is low. Lesser amounts are available in whole grains, dairy products, fortified breakfast cereals, dark chocolate, nuts, and seeds. Zinc lozenges are also widely available in drug and food stores.

Having diabetes may cause you to lose more zinc through your urine when your blood glucose level is high. Since zinc plays a role in the synthesis, storage, and secretion of insulin from pancreatic beta cells, a deficiency may interfere with your normal release of insulin if you have type 2 diabetes. Furthermore, some diabetic complications, such as changes to the retina in the eye, may be related to increased oxidative stress associated with decreases in zinc.

Taking zinc supplements containing even 25 mg per day may interfere with the absorption of other minerals, such as copper and iron, even though the upper intake level for zinc via supplements is currently set at 40 mg daily. Doses of over 100 mg daily may actually increase the bad cholesterol in your blood while decreasing the good type, as well as contribute to the development of anemia. Also, the potential benefits to the immune system from zinc are not evident with large doses (which may actually worsen your immune function). Take a low-dose supplement only if you can't sustain adequate zinc levels through your diet.

Spice up your food (and health) with cinnamon

Cinnamon has recently been investigated for its potential antidiabetic effects. It contains bioactive phenols (chemical compounds) that act as phytonutrients, and at least one study has shown that taking 1 to 6 grams of cinnamon per day may reduce your blood glucose, triglycerides (circulating blood fats), LDL, and total cholesterol if you have type 2 diabetes. One gram is about the equivalent of one-half tea-spoon of ground cinnamon. You can also get it in capsule form. If you plan on taking supplemental cinnamon for a long period of time, use a supplement made from a water extract of the spice, as regular cin-namon also contains coumarins that can thin the blood, an effect that you may not desire if you already take aspirin or other blood thinners.

What about Pycnogenol as an antioxidant?

Pycnogenol is an antioxidant supplement made from pine bark that contains a group of bioflavonoids called procyanidines. This compound is a potent antioxidant with several mechanisms of ac-tion. It may help preserve eye function in people with diabetic retinopathy, improve blood flow through small blood vessels, help lower blood pressure, and improve erectile function in men. Pro-cyanidines are also found in peanut skins, grape seed, and witch hazel bark. If you choose to supplement with Pycnogenol, the sug-gested dose is 50 mg three times a day.

Better memory and health with gingko biloba?

Gingko biloba is purported to restore memory, among other things. It has been used medicinally for thousands of years and is currently one of the top selling herbs in the United States. Many herbs and supple-ments, including this one, have not been thoroughly tested, and its safety and effectiveness have not been proven with regard to all of its supposed benefits (such as improvement in diabetic retinopathy). An-other problem with taking this herbal preparation is that various brands may be made differently and with variable ingredients, even within the same brand. If you do choose to take a supplement, take only the leaves and avoid the seeds as they are potentially toxic and could impact your blood sugar. So monitor them carefully when you begin taking the herb. Finally, avoid supplementing with it if you are already taking an anticlotting medication or will be having surgery in the near future because it does appear to lower your clotting ability.

Gamma-linolenic acid and nerve pain

Another nutritional supplement for people with diabetes is an omega-6 fatty acid, gamma-linolenic acid (GLA), believed to be the active ingredient found in the plant seed oils of evening primrose, black currant, borage, and fungal oils, along with spirulina (blue-green algae). A small number of studies have suggested that GLA may be helpful in treating diabetic neuropathy resulting in pain or numbness, and it may act by reducing inflammation. However, this compound may also lower clotting ability so check with your doctor about supplementing with it if you are taking aspirin, Coumadin, or other blood thinners. The currently recommended daily dose for people with diabetes who wish to supplement with GLA is 480 mg.

Capsaicin in hot chili peppers to the rescue?

Another herbal preparation is capsaicin, found in hot chili peppers (cayenne, red, African chilies, and Tabasco peppers), which has been used to treat painful nerve damage in diabetes. In the form of cayenne peppers, capsaicin has been used with variable success in folk medicine since the 1800s to treat colds, allergies, arthritis, and even hemorrhoids. Nowadays, you can buy it in over-the-counter topical salves (capsaicin creams), which have been approved by the Food and Drug Administration for treating chronic pain. While capsaicin is sometimes useful in relieving pain from diabetic neuropathy, its success is variable and can even make pain worse for some people. If you have painful diabetic neuropathy, one of these may help relieve the pain, but consult your doctor before trying it.

Recently capsaicin was reported as curing type 1 diabetes in mice in a study in which researchers injected the mice with a chemical transmitter of pain, substance P, which worked in concert with the capsaicin to improve nerve function in the pancreas and restore insulin production. In principle, it should also work to restore insulin production in people with type 2 diabetes. Whether this approach will work in humans remains to be seen, but it gives us hope that alternate approaches may work to stop the diabetes epidemic in its tracks.

What about ginseng, berberine, and bitter melon?

The herbal diabetes remedies that have been tried for diabetes are too numerous to list in this book, but there are a few more that you may find interesting. Three herbs in particular, ginseng, rhizoma coptidis (berberine, the major active compound), and bitter melon, have been used in Chinese medicine for centuries. Ginseng extracts made from root, rootlet, berry, and leaf of *Panax quinquefolium* (American ginseng) and *Panax ginseng* (Asian ginseng) may lower blood sugar levels, improve insulin action, help protect the pancreatic beta cells, and act as an antioxidant compound. Similarly, berberine from *Rhizoma coptidis* is used to help lower blood sugar, body weight, and blood fat levels. Finally, bitter melon or bitter gourd (*Momordica charantia*) is purported to reduce blood glucose and fats, protect beta cells, enhance insulin action, and reduce oxidative damage. Although evidence from animals and humans supports the therapeutic activities of these herbal medicines, multicenter large-scale clinical trials have not been conducted to evaluate their efficacy and safety, so use them with caution if you choose to. The same goes for other

---

Finding the Nutrient Content of Foods and Supplements

One way to eat healthier is to select foods that are nutrient dense—high in nutrient content for a given number of calories. You can easily check the nutrient content of any food on the USDA's website (www.nal.usda .gov/fnic/foodcomp) by clicking the Search the Nutrient Database button. The list of foods encompasses more than 6,000 items, and each is analyzed for nearly 120 separate nutrients. By choosing the Nutrient Lists option, you can also search for single nutrients within foods, making it easier to identify foods high in desirable nutrients like calcium, iron, fiber, and certain phytonutrients, as well as less desired elements like calories and saturated fat.

As for supplements, the metabolic effects of most nutrients are frequently synergistic with others found in whole foods in their natural state, which you aren't likely to get when you ingest a particular nutrient in supplement form. For more information on the nutrient content of supplements and foods, access any of several government websites, including the USDA site listed above, the Clinical Center for the NIH (www .cc.nih.gov/ccc/supplements) site, or the FDA's Center for Food Safety and Applied Nutrition site (www.cfsan.fda.gov/~dms/supplmnt.html).

---

supplemental foods, such as white vinegar, which is purported to lower fasting blood sugar when taken in the evening.

The health benefits of adequate protein, soy, and whey

In addition to helping with weight loss, most foods containing a significant amount of protein have a lower glycemic effect as proteins are metabolized more slowly than carbohydrates (usually within three to four hours). As long as your kidneys are functioning normally, taking in a diet that gets 30 to 40 percent of calories from protein, with a lower intake of carbs and fats, assists with glycemic control, weight loss, and weight maintenance. Pick high-quality sources of protein such as lean meats, soy products, legumes, and fish, all of which are lower in saturated and total fat and calories.

A diet rich in soy protein appears to have a lasting beneficial effect for people with type 2 diabetes. In a recent study published in *Diabetes Care*, researchers found that soy protein consumption had a significant positive impact on cardiovascular risk factors and kidney-related biomarkers among type 2 diabetic individuals with existing kidney disease. These patients were studied after consuming a diet consisting of 35 percent textured soy protein, 35 percent animal protein, and 30 percent vegetable protein for four years. Compared with controls, subjects who ate soy protein showed significantly lower levels of fasting blood sugar, total cholesterol, LDL cholesterol, and triglycerides, along with low levels of C-reactive protein (an indicator of inflammation) and urinary markers of kidney disease.

Eating enough protein in general—not just soy protein—is important as you age. The major building blocks of protein are amino acids. As you get older, your body may need a greater protein intake compared to when you were younger in order to form, maintain, and repair protein structures in the body like muscles. For example, adults over fifty may need about 1.1 grams of protein per kilogram (kg) of body weight (1 kilogram equals 2.2 pounds), while younger adults minimally require 0.8 grams per kg. All regularly exercising adults, regardless of the type of exercise or age, need more protein than this minimal amount (usually 1.1 to 1.6 grams per kg).

We also now know that certain amino acid compounds are especially important for maintaining muscle strength over time. Although well established in weight lifters and other power athletes for gaining muscle mass, creatine supplements taken in combination with doing resistance training may increase your strength gains arising from training. Similarly, an essential amino acid found mainly in whey protein derived from cow's milk called leucine is an important building block for muscles of which it is essential to consume adequate amounts. Although getting these compounds through your foods is still the preferred method, both can be found as dietary supplements in stores.

Are you deficient in carnitine?

A relatively new finding is that many people with diabetes are deficient in carnitine, which is produced by your body from amino acids (protein building blocks). This compound is important because it transports fats into the cell's powerhouse (the mitochondria) to be oxidized to produce energy. "Carnitine" is a generic term to describe L-carnitine, acetyl-L-carnitine, and propionyl-L-carnitine, but only the L-carnitine form, the one active in your body, is found in food. If your body doesn't produce enough (as is often the case in people with diabetes), then you must get more in your diet. It is important because it increases your insulin action and is essential for metabolizing fats and carbohydrates. Supplementation with carnitine can improve insulin sensitivity by decreasing fat levels and glucose in blood.

Carnitine supplementation may help lessen some diabetic complications as well. In a study of 1,200 diabetic patients, researchers found that treatment of type 1 or type 2 diabetes with acetyl-L-carnitine (500 mg or 1,000 mg doses daily) for a year relieved diabetes-related nerve pain in feet and sensation of vibration there. Thus it may actually help delay progression of neuropathic pain related to diabetes or reduce its severity.

If your body makes enough, you won't need to take any supplements or even worry about consuming any carnitine naturally in foods. If you're deficient, though—as most diabetic individuals and anyone undergoing renal dialysis are—then you can find it in meat, fish, poultry, and milk. It is most concentrated in whey protein found in dairy products. It is also safe to take it as a supplement of L-carnitine (the biologically active form) or acetyl-L-carnitine, both of which are sold online and in health food stores, usually in 500 or 1,000 mg doses.

Nonprescription treatments for diabetic complications

For annoying but not potentially fatal complications like frozen joints, trigger fingers, and other tendonitis, the best solutions vary. Frozen shoulder (known medically as adhesive capsulitis) can often be treated with trigger point massage and physical therapy. For others, frozen joints (which includes shoulders primarily, but also hips) slow them down for a while, but don't knock them out for good. Trigger fingers that result in excessive curling can be treated surgically, which many people with diabetes have had to undergo on more than one digit. For other joint or tendon inflammation, prophylactic use of anti-inflammatory medications like ibuprofen and aspirin may work to control pain and stiffness before they limit your activities. Exercising regularly and using the full range of motion around your joints may help prevent some of these occurrences.

Many people with diabetes have turned to herbal remedies and supplements to try to control symptoms of peripheral neuropathy, which can result in pain in your feet and hands and numbness. Some individuals swear by omega-3 fatty acid supplements, not just to counteract the effects of peripheral nerve damage but also to treat joint pain related to tendonitis, along with glucosamine supplements. Another herbal treatment for neuropathy is quercetin, one of the natural phytonutrients from plants called flavonoids that others have used to reverse the numbness in their legs and feet.

Alpha lipoic acid (LA) may combat several complications by inhibiting the formation of plaque in coronary arteries, lowering blood fat levels, and reducing systemic inflammation and possibly weight gain when taken in large doses. It also may reduce the symptoms of neuropathy in the feet and hands (e.g., burning, pain, and numbness) when taken as a supplement, as may supplemental vitamin D and acetyl-L-carnitine.

Others have tried taking a natural cocktail of antioxidants, including LA, borage oil (high in GLA, also found in evening primrose oil), benfotiamine (a derivative of thiamine, or vitamin B1), and vitamin C. In fact, one of Dr. Sheri's research colleagues, Dr. Aaron Vinik, a renowned neuropathy specialist, has actually created his own formulation, which he now markets as NutriNerve. It contains varying amounts of LA, GLA, and benfotiamine.

A recent study suggested that a large number of alternate treatments might offer relief from complications like painful neuropathy. In addition to the ones mentioned, others include folate (a B vitamin), myo-inositol, omega-3 and omega-6 fatty acids, L-glutamine, taurine, zinc, magnesium, chromium, and St. John's Wort. You can also get supplements like Foltx and Folgard, both of which contain combinations of B vitamins like folate, vitamin B6, and vitamin B12 to treat neuropathy pain. Try taking a B-complex vitamin if you can't afford these supplements.

Some individuals have tried topical creams, such as ones containing capsaicin or lidocaine, to temporarily reduce painful episodes in feet and hands. You can make your own capsaicin cream by mixing one to two teaspoons of cayenne pepper into cold cream and applying it to affected areas. If you do so, take care to cover your hands with disposable plastic gloves first.

In an interesting trial treatment, honey was applied topically to diabetic foot ulcers. In one case study, an individual with nonhealing ulcers on his toes and heels was instructed to apply a heavy coating of honey on a gauze pad, which he taped over the affected areas of his feet and reapplied daily. Within six to twelve months of doing this regularly, all of the ulcers had healed on their own without antibiotics, even though all previous treatment attempts had failed miserably. This healing effect has been attributed to a natural antibacterial quality of honey. You'll have sticky feet during this treatment, though. Some individuals have also spent time in decompression chambers (normally used for scuba divers who ascend too rapidly and get decompression sickness) to help their foot and lower limb diabetic ulcers heal. In the chamber, the pressure is increased during a treatment session, which apparently increases circulation to affected areas and speeds up healing.

In general, antioxidants like LA are believed to be integrally involved in the prevention of many diabetic complications such as cataracts, which result at least partially from deficient glutathione levels leading to a faulty antioxidant defense system within the lens of your eye. Nutrients such as LA, vitamins E and C, and selenium can increase your levels of glutathione and its activity, allowing for better protection of your eyes and other tissues. Taking too much of these disease-fighting compounds can be counterproductive, though, as almost all antioxidants have been shown to have the opposite effect when taken in unnaturally large doses. Don't go overboard when taking them or any prescribed medications. LA may improve blood sugar control, so if you are taking medications to lower your blood sugar, such as metformin (Glucophage) or glyburide (DiaBeta, Glynase), do so under the supervision of a physician or other qualified health professional and carefully monitor your glucose levels.

A final note: Let your physician know about any herbal remedies you're using since they can potentially interact with prescribed medications and cause bad side effects. The scientific findings about such herbal and vitamin remedies are not conclusive currently, so Dr. Leo is hesitant to officially prescribe any of these for his patients.

CHAPTER 4: *En pocas palabras*

Certain herbal remedies, foods, or dietary supplements may help your diabetes control and overall health, particularly antioxidants like alpha lipoic acid; many of the B vitamins; vitamins C, D, and E; minerals like magnesium, zinc, and chromium; and natural foods containing capsaicin, soy, carnitine, cinnamon, Pycnogenol, gamma-linolenic acid, and more. Learn the potential benefits of each one and choose your supplements with care to optimize your health. Be sure to inform your doctor about any herbal or dietary supplements you take, especially if you take prescribed medications for your diabetes or other health problems, to avoid potential interactions.

CHAPTER 5

Moving More for Your Body, Heart, and Mind

In general, Latino culture encourages good eating but little exercise. Some Latinos perceive that media stars and other celebrities are excessively thin because they exercise too much, when in reality exercise should be required because of its many health benefits. From a metabolic standpoint, it's always better to be fit, no matter how much you weigh. Physical activity of almost any type enhances your insulin action and makes diabetes easier to control, and it may even enhance your insulin production as long as you have functioning beta cells to make insulin in your pancreas. Regular exercise also lowers your risk of premature death, heart disease, certain types of cancers (colon, for example), anxiety and depression, osteoporosis, and severe arthritic symptoms. It even helps you sleep better, which is important because sleeping too little (e.g., five hours or less a night) has been linked with an increased incidence of diabetes and being overweight.

Regardless of what type of exercise works best for you or how you get motivated to do it regularly, it is helpful to understand how activity affects your blood glucose levels. In this chapter we'll suggest ways to get started moving more and what types of activity to include as part of a healthy, diabetes-controlling lifestyle. In addition, you will learn what effect being active has on losing weight and keeping it off, what you need to know about exercising safely with diabetes or its complications, and other exercise-related facts that are important to being active.

Latino-specific barriers to being active

Most people have excuses for not being more physically active. What will it take to get Latinos in particular moving more? One study of Mexican Americans with diabetes looked at just that. Apparently participants were more motivated to exercise when they had family support, and the sense of well-being they got from doing it also acted as a motivator. Barriers to exercising included physical pain, depression, excess body weight, unsafe neighborhoods, inadequate exercise facilities, and a perceived lack of time. They stated that if they could use a gym or fitness center at a low cost, they would be more inclined to work out regularly, especially if the facility were family oriented and close to home with classes led by bilingual instructors. Finally, their preferred mode of exercise was walking (and gardening), especially with friends and family members.

Exercise releases glucose-raising hormones

When you begin to exercise, your body immediately responds by releasing hormones that increase your blood glucose levels, which must be maintained for your brain and nervous system to function properly. Your body has a relatively limited supply of glucose stored in muscles and liver as glycogen and far less glucose circulating in your bloodstream. Carbohydrates are the primary fuel your body uses during exercise. The hormones released during exercise send a signal to your liver, which replaces what your muscles use by breaking down glycogen to form glucose or by making new glucose from lactic acid or other precursors. Another pancreatic hormone, glucagon, has the most direct effect on the liver with regard to releasing enough glucose. Adrenaline (epinephrine) raises your heart rate and signals your exercising muscles to break down glycogen and some fat as well. At the same time, your body lowers its insulin levels to keep your muscles from taking up too much glucose. Other hormones, such as norepinephrine, growth hormone, and cortisol, effectively redistribute blood and provide other fuels to working muscles and the liver during physical activity.

When your blood glucose level is higher than normal, such as after you eat a meal loaded with higher-GI carbohydrates, exercise usually helps lower it. However, depending on how fast you move, how hard you work out, and how long you are active, exercise can lower, maintain, or even raise blood glucose levels. While long-duration activities almost always lower it, weight lifting or other intense activities can cause your glucose-raising hormones to produce more sugar than your body needs and raise your blood glucose levels. This effect is usually short-lived, and blood glucose will typically return to normal within an hour or two. You can also reduce or prevent this effect by doing ten to twenty minutes of easier (aerobic) exercise like slow walking afterward, which will have a glucose-lowering effect.

At rest, your body uses a mix of about 60 percent fat and 40 percent carbohydrate (with insignificant protein use), but during exercise, carbohydrates supply the majority of the fuel, particularly when you work out harder. Depletion of both your muscle glycogen and blood glucose is inevitable if you're active for many hours. Your body can also use fat, but fat contributes most during mild- to moderate-intensity workouts. During recovery from exercise, though, when your body is restocking depleted fuels, fat use predominates.

Exercising helps control your blood sugar

Having insulin in your bloodstream is the only way you can lower your blood sugar at rest. During exercise, muscle contractions force glucose out of your blood and into your muscles without relying on insulin (via a separate mechanism). Muscular activity essentially gives you an alternate way to lower your blood sugar that does not depend on having enough insulin or being insulin sensitive. Exercise actually comes close to acting like a dose of insulin (released by your pancreas or injected) with respect to its glucose-lowering effects.

Your muscles make up about 40 percent of your body weight, but they can take up and store close to 80 percent of any glucose load ingested with carbohydrate intake. By enhancing your muscles' capacity to take up glucose with or without insulin, exercise comes closer than anything else to counterbalancing excess food intake or reduced insulin action, which both cause high blood sugar. You will be able to eat more carbohydrate and process it more effectively following hard or prolonged workouts than at any other time. The only potential downside of exercise's ability to stimulate glucose uptake on its own is that if your insulin levels are too high when you're exercising (particularly due to injected insulin, if you take any), your sugars can drop rapidly in response to the additive effects of insulin and muscular activity.

Simply taking more steps will use up blood glucose and keep your levels lower during the day. Sedentary, insulin-resistant middle-aged adults engaging in thirty minutes of moderate walking three to seven days per week for six months succeeded in reversing their pre-diabetic state, even without changing their diet or losing weight. Similarly, in older adults, low- to moderate-intensity "walking" on minitrampolines for twenty to forty minutes four days per week over a four-month period enhanced their glucose uptake without any additional insulin release or loss of abdominal fat.

Exercise prolongs your increased insulin action for at least a brief period afterward

Your insulin action will be heightened most in the first couple of hours following an activity and diminish over time as your glycogen is replaced. When carbohydrate use is significant (as during thirty minutes of continuous moderate exercise), your blood glucose levels decrease during the activity, and then for two or more hours afterward, your muscles continue to take up more blood glucose with very little insulin. A single workout, particularly if prolonged or intense, can enhance your insulin action for twenty-four hours or more while glycogen stores in your muscles and liver are being replenished. Moreover, when your insulin works better, you need less of it to have the same or even a greater glucose-lowering effect. During this time, you will likely need less insulin to process carbohydrates that you eat. In addition, athletic muscles store less excess fat in them, which increases their responsiveness to insulin.

The duration of your daily physical activity is important to achieve and maintain heightened insulin action. Recent studies suggest that participating in almost three hours (170 minutes) of exercise per week at any intensity (easy, moderate, or hard) improves insulin action more than if you accumulate only two hours (120 minutes) weekly. The length of your physical activity appears to be more important for blood glucose control than how hard you work out. Your blood sugar will be easier to control if you move around as much as possible, even when you're not actually exercising.

Try walking instead of sitting

Researchers have found that overweight people sit over two hours a day longer than leaner ones, which is the caloric equivalent of about 350 calories per day or 36 pounds in a year. Just staying on your feet more can have a beneficial effect on your body weight. We used to believe that exercise had to be vigorous to bestow meaningful health benefits, but a study conducted at Harvard found that, for adult women at least, moderate walking decreases the risk of developing diabetes as effectively as more vigorous activities do.

Additional walking can be added into your daily routine in myriad ways, including walking around when you talk on the phone, taking the stairs instead of the elevator, walking up and down escalators (instead of standing on them), changing the channels on your TV without the remote control, washing dishes, and doing yard work and gardening. You can also walk around for five minutes after every half hour of being sedentary, or at least stand up. For better health, you need to expend those extra calories through physical activity in any way you can. Increase the number of steps that you take during the day and add in planned walks whenever you can.

The benefits of greater activity are almost endless. If you have type 2 diabetes and increase your aerobic activity by thirty-eight minutes per day (the equivalent of walking an extra 4,400 steps a day, or about 2.2 miles), you'll likely experience a lowering of your blood glucose, total cholesterol, triglycerides (blood fats), and blood pressure, even if you don't lose weight. You will also have a lower risk of heart disease and stroke and likely reduce your medical expenses.

MARILYN GARCIA
A Latina living well with type 1 diabetes
for more than fifty years

Marilyn Garcia's father is Hispanic (from Spain) but her mother is not. Type 1 diabetes entered her life when she was a young child, but she has lived well with it for fifty-one out of her fifty-seven years. She remembers having classic symptoms of type 1 diabetes before she was diagnosed with it, such as urinating a lot. No one else in her family had this type of diabetes (which is not an unusual phenomenon).

A lawyer practicing in Los Angeles, Marilyn believes that regularly monitoring her blood sugar is important to her doing well with diabetes. "I don't live a perfect life," she admits, "but I've tried to be as diligent as I can about monitoring and not getting discouraged." She also tries to look on the bright side of having diabetes. "All experiences have their positive side," she remarks. "I think I became a lawyer because having diabetes helps me keep track of time, which is a good trait to have when you practice law."

She also refuses to think of herself as being different because of her disease. During law school at Yale, she made friends with the first blind student going through the curriculum. She says, "I wanted to be treated like I was normal, just like he did. I didn't baby him like everyone else did. I think having a disease like diabetes makes you empathize with others in ways that others can't." As for staying positive about her own health, if she ever has to be admitted for a hospital stay for any reason, she views the hospital as an "interesting place to visit" instead of a place to be feared.

One of her keys to success is closely watching her diet. She has focused on eating healthy foods for years, and she thinks she is pretty good at figuring out what foods have in them and how much insulin she needs to give herself to cover them. Living in the United States, she enjoys having access to food labels that help her make these decisions. "I think it's great that we have food labels on the back of all consumer products. Seeing them makes it like a formula for me to manage my diabetes. I look at the number of carbs, and it makes figuring out the insulin dose a no-brainer."

Marilyn also feels that having access to a good diabetes physician is important. "I have a pretty good doctor, and I trust his judgment. I leave it up to him to recommend new things I should try." She appreciates that sometimes even when you think you know what you are doing, you need a professional perspective from someone who has the knowledge to help you adjust your insulin or your medications. Yet she has enough knowledge to manage diabetes most of the time on her own, which she had to do on many occasions when she was pregnant with both of her children. She realizes that for many in the Latino community, physicians are in a position of authority and people are a bit intimidated by that. She chooses instead to view a physician as a team player, just one of the group that helps her manage her diabetes effectively, and she suggests that others do the same.

With regard to being physically active, she remarks, "I don't like to exercise, and I haven't since day one with diabetes." Since learning about its beneficial effects on her blood sugar control, though, she now walks three miles at a time three days a week. "I know being active helps. When I go on vacation in Europe and walk around all day long, my blood glucose stays absolutely perfect. If I could just walk around Europe all the time, I'd be in great shape," she laughs. She can't be on vacation all the time, though, so in her daily life, she just tries to move around her office when she can.

Move more throughout the day

There's so much more to being physically active than just doing planned exercise sessions. Incorporate more movement into your life any way you can. Standing, talking, and fidgeting use up extra calories and can make a difference in your body weight and blood glucose control. Just adding a dozen steps here and there while doing household chores, yard work, or errands, along with standing, making extra

Tips for Adding in More Unstructured Exercise

- Add as many additional steps as possible (a minimum of 2,000) every day by walking whenever and wherever you can.
- Whenever you have ten free minutes, walk around instead of sitting down—or at least stand up.
- Get up and move around for a few minutes after every thirty minutes of a sedentary activity.
- Always take the stairs instead of the elevator or escalator.
- Do physical chores around the house, such as cleaning, sweeping, mopping, vacuuming, and washing dishes (even if you have a dishwasher).
- Do some gardening, rake leaves in the yard, or shovel snow.
- Go shopping for groceries or window-shopping at the nearest mall.
- Put on some music and dance around your house.
- Take salsa or other dance classes that fit into your Latino lifestyle.
- Set up a basketball hoop in your driveway or walk to the nearest neighborhood school and use those.
- Take the dog out for a daily walk—it needs exercise too!
- Walk around while talking on the telephone instead of sitting down.
- Hide the remotes for the TV, stereo, and other devices.
- Walk in place, dance, move around, or even just stand up while watching TV—at least during the commercial breaks.
- Limit your TV and home computer use to no more than two hours per day, or at least reduce your use by a minimum of thirty minutes daily.

arm movements, stretching, and other general body movement, can easily add up to a substantial amount of energy expended over the course of the day and can prevent insulin resistance and weight gain. In fact, doing any regular physical activity during your leisure time decreases your risk of diabetes and other health problems, even if it's salsa or merengue dancing or other fun activities.

All exercise you do during the day counts. Participating in intense activities (such as jogging) is not necessary for optimal health and fitness. Pick your favorite leisure-time activity—be it golfing, gardening, mowing the lawn, walking the dog, salsa dancing, or social walking with your family—and do it for a total of thirty to forty-five minutes per day (for as little as 10 minutes at a time). Even if your fitness level is not increased much, your overall health will benefit. Your goal is simply to be as physically active as possible during the day to maximize caloric expenditure and blood glucose use. The more, the better, so think of creative ways to add more movement into each and every day. *¡No problema!*

Include some planned aerobic activities

Leisure-time and other unstructured activities are great to incorporate into your improved lifestyle, but you likely should also add in some planned activity to maximize your fitness and diabetes control. For instance, stretching and other flexibility activities are important in limiting flexibility losses as you age, although they don't lower your blood glucose much. As already noted, prolonged aerobic workouts generally lower blood glucose levels, but resistance training provides additional benefits.

Aerobic (or cardio) exercise gets your heart working harder. As your blood is pumped faster, it must be oxygenated in less time as it passes through your lungs, which in turn quickens your breathing. Consequently aerobic exercise strengthens your heart and boosts good cholesterol levels. Lower-impact aerobic exercises include easy walking, swimming, cycling, tai chi, and the like. Higher-impact aerobic exercise includes running, tennis, aerobic dance classes, and salsa and other dancing.

The surgeon general has recommended moderate amounts of daily aerobic physical activity for people of all ages, including thirty minutes of moderate activities (like brisk walking) or shorter sessions—fifteen to twenty minutes—of more intense exercise, including jogging or playing basketball. Ideally, structured aerobic exercise programs should involve activities that allow you to move your whole body over the greatest distance possible to maximize your energy use. Although walking and jogging fall into this category, most overweight adults will find jogging and running either too difficult or simply not fun. Of course, engaging in even more total physical activity may offer you additional benefits, but only up to a point. The incidence of activity-related injuries, such as inflamed tendons (tendonitis) and stress fractures in bones, rises dramatically when you do more than sixty to ninety minutes of moderate or hard exercise daily.

Brisk walking is likely the best medicine for both the prevention and treatment of type 2 diabetes and for your overall health, and it's more sustainable as a lifelong activity than many others. Try tricking yourself into walking by incorporating it into other activities, such as walking farther than you need to when you shop. Walking can be the gateway to more vigorous exercise, which can further increase your overall health benefits. Your self-confidence may improve once you start a walking program, which may lead you to additional physical activities, including ballroom or other Latino-type dancing, cycling, or low-impact aerobics classes. Remember to take advantage of any strong physical attributes that you have, such as stronger legs from carrying around your extra body weight.

If you're currently sedentary and overweight, you may resist exercising. Ease into being more active by taking small steps in that direction. Do activities that don't require you to carry around your full body weight, such as swimming, classes in a swimming pool, seated exercises, stationary cycling, stretching, and light resistance training. For the first two, fat stored under the skin acts to insulate you and keep you warmer in the pool, where you lose body heat faster than in air. Just walking or moving in the water, which additionally helps hide your figure and lower your resistance to doing exercise in public, is a good choice. Seated exercises or stationary cycling also reduce stress on your lower limb joints.

As you gradually become more fit, you may find yourself trying activities that you were previously incapable of doing. What about salsa or other Latino dancing? It counts as aerobic exercise, and you can enjoy yourself while doing it. Even when you're watching TV, you can walk in place or climb onto an elliptical trainer, treadmill, or stationary cycle and get some more exercise. Pick the exercises that work best for you and your unique preferences and lifestyle.

Chair and Other Exercise Workouts on DVD (or CD)

A wide selection of videos and DVDs demonstrating various physical activities, including dancing and exercise routines with a Latino flair as well as exercise done in a chair or wheelchair, are available from a variety of sources. You can find materials for aerobic workouts, strength training, flexibility moves, yoga, and other types of exercise. In addition to finding them at local sporting-goods stores and national chains, there are many online sources to peruse for workout DVDs. Some of the more promising ones (for various fitness levels) follow:

- *Viva! Latin Rhythm Workout* (2000)
- *Quenia Ribeiro's Dance Today! Samba: Active Lifestyle Makeover* (2006)
- *Vanessa Isaac's Samba Party Workout 1: Brazilian Rhythm Celebration* (2005)
- *Vanessa Isaac's Brazilian Dance Workout* (2003)
- *World Dance Workout: Bellydance, Bollywood, Salsa, Samba, Flamenco* (2006)

- *Tru2Form: Latin Dance Workouts* (2006; available in English and Spanish)
- *Zumba DVD Collection* (2008; available at www.zumba.com)
- *Leslie Sansone's Walk Away the Pounds: Complete In-Home Walking System* (2007)
- *Senior Resistance Bands Exercise DVD for Strength and Fitness* (2005)
- *Beginners Fitness/Exercise DVD with Light Weights: Women, Over 50, Baby Boomers Fitness and Easy Weight Loss Exercise* (2005)
- *Chair Aerobics for Everyone* (2006)
- *Jodi Stolove's Chair Dancing Through the Decades* (2004) and *Chair Dancing around the World* (2004) (find all her CDs at www.chairdancing.com)
- *Bob Klein's Chair Exercises for Seniors* (Zookinesis) (2004)
- *Sunrise Tai Chi* (2005)
- *Chair Aerobics for Everyone: Chair Tai Chi* (2007)
- *Yoga Therapy Prescriptions: 60 Health Restorative Sequences* (2008)
- *Chair and Standing Routines: Ageless Yoga, Volume 1, Great for Seniors and for People Unable to Sit on the Ground* (2006)
- *Stronger Seniors Fitness Program: 2 DVD Stretch and Strength Chair Exercise for Seniors* (2007)
- You can also download free audio or video music tracks from *Movimiento por Su Vida* (*Movement for Your Life*) from www.cdc.gov/diabetes/ndep/movimiento.htm, or order this music CD, which features six original songs with empowering messages and strong Latin rhythms.

Add in some weights for greater insulin power

In addition to walking or other aerobic activities, you can further improve your insulin action and blood glucose control by doing weight training. Muscle fibers run the spectrum from being very aerobic (slow-twitch fibers) to being mainly recruited for heavy lifting or near-maximal exercise (fast-twitch fibers); all types of fibers can exist within a single muscle. For easy work, you use only the very aerobic (slow) fibers in the muscles you're using. However, if you increase your workload, you'll be recruiting not just the slow ones, but also some of the intermediate-speed fibers. A maximal weight lift (or all-out sprint) recruits all of these plus your very fastest fibers, which are capable of producing the most power in the shortest amount of time.

Why is it so important to recruit all of your muscle fibers? Like so many systems in your body, if you don't use them, you lose them over time. This is especially true when it comes to muscle fibers and muscle mass. Anyone past the age of twenty-five is slowly losing muscle mass, which in turn reduces your glycogen storage capacity and lowers your insulin action. To keep your insulin working well and your diabetes under control, you need to retain as much of your muscle mass as possible—and even gain muscle if you can. For example, newly diagnosed type 2 diabetic men who did sixteen weeks of progressive resistance training (the resistance lifted was increased over time) twice weekly gained muscle mass, lost body fat (particularly intra-abdominal), and enhanced their insulin action, even though they were eating 15 percent more calories.

Similarly, in people with type 2 diabetes, four to six weeks of moderate-intensity (40 to 50 percent of maximal) resistance training improved their insulin sensitivity by 48 percent without significant changes in their body fat or muscle mass. Although you're preventing additional loss of muscle with training, be forewarned that it takes more than six weeks to experience noticeable gains in the amount of muscle you have; you'll be able to tell when it happens because you will see more definition to your muscles when you are working them.

Among older Hispanic adults with diabetes, resistance exercise for sixteen weeks improved their muscle quality, whole-body insulin action, and blood sugar control, while lowering inflammation that causes cardiovascular disease. If you're an older, type 2 diabetic woman, the combination of aerobic and resistance training may afford even greater improvements in your insulin action, increased muscle mass, and a more significant decrease in your abdominal fat than aerobic training alone. Resistance training can bestow extra health benefits, such as a higher metabolism, greater self-esteem, feelings of accomplishment, and greater strength in as little as one to two weeks (from neural changes that occur before increases in muscle size). Major strength gains are possible even if you train as infrequently as one day a week, although two to three nonconsecutive days a week are recommended. Strength gains are also the key to preventing injuries, particularly from falling, which occurs more often as people age.

Interval training offers additional benefits

Doing more intense activities—even occasionally or intermittently—benefits diabetes control. A study involved people with type 2 diabetes walking over 10,000 steps a day; they began pick up the pace (PUP) training, which involved some faster-paced walking. They measured their usual walking speed (in steps taken per minute measured with a pedometer) and then began walking for thirty minutes, three times a week, at a pace that was only 10 percent higher than normal (a usual pace of 90 steps per minute would be upped to about 100 instead). Twelve weeks of PUP training for ninety minutes a week improved insulin action and increased the participants' fitness level since they get done sooner.

To get started with similar training and benefits, simply increase the intensity of your exercise for short periods of time (thereby doing interval training) to gain more from it. When you're walking, speed up slightly for a short distance (such as between two light poles or mailboxes) before slowing back down to your original pace. Continue to include these short, faster intervals during your walks or other activities, and lengthen them out to last two to five minutes each (or even up to thirty minutes, as was done in the PUP study) as you can. You will end up more fit, use more calories, feel more tired when you finish, and may even find that your general walking speed has increased due to the extra conditioning.

Get the Most out of Your Exercise Training

- Move more all day long to build your overall endurance.
- Alternate hard and easy workout days to maximize results and minimize injuries.
- Intersperse occasional faster intervals into each activity.
- Do at least one longer workout each week to build greater endurance.
- Focus on spending a greater amount of time being active (as opposed to worrying about your workout intensity) to benefit blood glucose levels.
- If your workouts are short, work harder to use more muscle glycogen.
- Include resistance training as often as possible, preferably two to three days per week.
- Cross train by doing a variety of activities for greater fitness, better motivation, and injury prevention.
- Use a full range of motion around your joints during all activities, if possible.
- Rest at least one day a week (to allow your body to fully repair itself), but avoid taking off more than two days in a row so that your insulin action doesn't decrease too much.

Stretch to keep your joints mobile

Doing stretching or yoga several times a week is an important part of being active; working on your flexibility helps prevent injuries and is doubly important for anyone with diabetes. Everyone loses flexibility over time, but an elevated blood glucose level by itself can speed up this loss by binding to joint structures (like collagen) and making them more brittle and less flexible. Less flexibility leads to a reduced range of motion for your joints, an increased likelihood of orthopedic injuries, and a greater risk of developing joint-related problems often associated with diabetes, such as diabetic frozen shoulder, tendonitis, trigger finger, and carpal tunnel syndrome. Regular stretching and using the full range of motion around each of your joints can help prevent these problems.

Expending calories through exercise is the key to a healthy weight

There are other reasons to be more physically active that have less to do with diabetes and insulin action and more to do with changing your body weight and shape for the better. A new study showed that overeating, rather than the obesity it causes, is the trigger for developing health problems like metabolic syndrome and diabetes—ones that involve insulin resistance, fatty liver, heart disease, and more. This study is among the first to recognize that weight gain is an early symptom of metabolic syndrome, prediabetes, and diabetes rather than a direct cause. The spillover of excess fat into organs like the liver or heart is what damages them, while depositing excess calories as fat in fat cells actually delays these harmful effects. For example, genetically altered mice whose fat cells can't expand when overfed develop metabolic syndrome very rapidly.

Even though excess body fat may not be the direct cause of most health problems, losing body fat or maintaining your body weight is a worthwhile goal in which exercise plays an important role. Regardless of how much weight you lose or don't lose by being active, regular physical activity can prevent you from developing type 2 diabetes in the first place or reverse prediabetes. Weight loss can also help control diabetes in many individuals, regardless of what type of diabetes they have. A new analysis of the Diabetes Prevention Program (designed to prevent type 2) published in *Diabetes Care* in 2006 found that weight loss is most directly correlated to a decreased risk of developing the disease. Participants' weight loss was predicted by how much exercise they did, and only the ones who continued to exercise after the trial ended maintained their new, lower body weights. Regular physical activity makes a huge difference in whether you will experience weight gain, maintenance, or loss, and the lifestyle behaviors that help you keep your weight down (like regular exercise) likely will benefit your diabetes control the most.

As discussed previously, visceral fat stored deep within your abdomen is the worst type of body fat with regard to diabetes control because it makes your insulin work less effectively. Luckily, both moderate aerobic exercise and resistance training (done even only twice a week) can result in losses of visceral fat that dieting alone doesn't cause, and you can be fit regardless of your body weight. You can also gain almost all of the associated health benefits of having a higher fitness level without struggling to lose weight and keep it off.

Furthermore, studies examining the effects of being fat, fit, or both on the risk of developing a debilitating illness or dying have found that as your weight increases, so does your risk of dying from heart disease or developing diabetes. However, the more physically fit you are, the lower your risk of dying from any cause. In other words, fat weight gain and unfitness are independent risk factors for heart disease, mortality, and diabetes. While it is still best to be fit and thin, being fit and fat is healthier than being thin and unfit. What you definitely don't want to be is fat and unfit.

Why exercise makes your body weight change more slowly

Exercise can't make your body weight go down faster than dieting alone. The weight that you lose through cutting back on calories consists of body fat, muscle mass, and water weight. Exercise causes you to retain and even gain some muscle mass, which is desirable given that muscle is sensitive to insulin and is a storehouse for carbohydrates and blood glucose. Muscle is denser than body fat and thus weighs more. Consequently you can lose fat while retaining or gaining muscle with exercise. Your weight on the scale may change very little (or even rise slightly at first), even though your body composition (total fat and muscle) is changing for the better.

If you feel you must weigh yourself frequently after you start an exercise program, keep these changes in mind. Better yet, focus on your waist and hip measurements and how loose your clothes are getting rather than your body weight. Never weigh yourself more than once a week, and always do it at the same time of day under similar circumstances (e.g., before eating breakfast). Even if exercising regularly doesn't make you lose all of the weight you want to, it can still prevent you from gaining weight while you lose fat and gain muscle.

Making lifestyle changes, such as including exercise as a part of your daily routine, is a much better method of both accomplishing better blood glucose control and losing weight than using supplemental insulin to improve overall diabetes control. When people with type 2 diabetes implement such changes, their diabetes control improves similarly to those who either have just begun using insulin or who implement the same lifestyle changes along with using insulin, and they offset some of the weight gain possible with supplemental insulin use. If you fail to maintain your lifestyle changes, though, your gains will be lost.

Does the time of day you exercise make a difference?

Your body experiences a transient state of insulin resistance first thing in the morning, which is when you have higher levels of cortisol and other hormones that helped your liver keep your blood sugar from dropping overnight. Exercising before breakfast may not have the glucose-lowering effect that you desire. In moderately hyperglycemic type 2 diabetic men treated with oral diabetic medications, one hour of moderate cycling caused their blood glucose levels to decrease minimally when they exercised before eating breakfast, but drop dramatically (down to normal) when exercising two hours after eating breakfast. Likely, it's best to eat (and take your diabetic medications) before exercising in the early morning if you want to lower your blood sugar levels. On the other hand, if you tend to drop too low during activities, exercising at that time of day may prevent low blood sugar. Moderate walking and similar exercises after dinner also help prevent postmeal spikes in blood sugar, more so than the same exercise done before a meal.

CHAPTER 5: *En pocas palabras*

For the treatment and prevention of type 2 diabetes, regular physical activity is a critical lifestyle choice that has not traditionally been popular among Latinos. Engaging family support for being more active is an effective motivational strategy, along with simply moving more each day, taking extra steps, and incorporating structured exercise that includes aerobics, resistance training, and stretching into your daily life. Being physically active is a key in managing body weight as well. Retaining and gaining muscle mass are also critical in improving your insulin action and diabetes control, which can only be accomplished with regular training.

CHAPTER 6

Learning How to Exercise Safely and Effectively

Despite the many benefits of physical activity (Chapter 5), it has a potential downside. In this chapter, we focus on what you need to know in order to exercise safely and effectively, even with preexisting health complications. To get the most out of your training, you'll want to learn how to avoid and treat low and high blood sugar, prevent dehydration, and work around any health concerns that you have. After reading this chapter, you will see that almost everyone can find an appropriate way to exercise.

Do you need to see your doctor before you start to exercise?

You probably don't need a checkup before engaging in low-intensity exercise like walking, but having one before you begin more vigorous workouts is a good idea. If you have more risk factors for heart disease (e.g., smoking, high cholesterol levels, family history of early

Get a Checkup First if You . . .

- Are planning on participating in moderate to strenuous activities, not just mild ones
- Are over thirty-five years of age
- Have been diagnosed with type 1 diabetes for more than fifteen years or type 2 diabetes for more than ten years
- Have heart disease, a strong family history of heart disease, or high cholesterol or lipid levels
- Have poor circulation in your feet or legs (or lower-leg pain while walking)
- Have diabetic eye disease (proliferative retinopathy), kidney problems (nephropathy), or nerve damage (numbness, burning, tingling, or loss of sensation in your feet and/or dizziness when going from sitting to standing)
- Have not consistently controlled your blood glucose levels
- Have any other concerns about exercising, including joint pain, arthritis, or other chronic health problems

heart attack, obesity, diabetes, etc.), your risk of having a heart attack or stroke during exercise is greater. You don't need to avoid exercise, particularly since doing regular moderate to vigorous activity can actually reduce your risk of a heart attack (even if you have already had one), but it's wise to realize your limitations.

Most people with type 2 diabetes would benefit from having a thorough medical exam prior to starting most exercise programs, including a physical exam, urinalysis, kidney function testing, serum lipid evaluation, electrolyte balance, and exercise stress testing. Such testing can screen for the presence of any diabetes-related complications, including heart, nerve, eye, and kidney disease. While having such health problems does not automatically preclude you from exercising, doing so safely and effectively with any of these complications may require special accommodations or precautions.

Learn how to exercise safely and effectively with diabetes

Exercise has a short-term effect on blood glucose levels, but there is a longer-lasting benefit as well—your insulin (natural or injected) will be more effective. With regular exercise, better insulin action will help lower your blood glucose levels and improve your diabetes control. However, preventing your blood sugar from getting too low or too high during exercise is critical to exercising safely and effectively, particularly if you use certain diabetic medications or insulin. Whenever you start doing new or different activities, plan on testing your blood sugar to determine how your body reacts, including before and after exercise and even during a workout. Some risk is present, especially if you have related health complications like neuropathy or heart disease. In the remainder of this chapter, you will learn how to exercise safely in spite of them.

What causes hypoglycemia, and what are its symptoms?

Hypoglycemia, usually defined as a blood glucose level lower than 65 mg/dl (3.6 mmol/L), requires immediate treatment when symptoms begin to occur. Keep a blood glucose meter handy to check your blood sugar regularly. It can be useful to check immediately after exercise, and then every thirty to sixty minutes for a couple of hours to determine what kind of lasting effect the exercise is having on you. Eat rapidly absorbed carbohydrates if your blood glucose level drops lower than you like or if you have symptoms of hypoglycemia.

Although mild or brisk walking generally allows your body to use some fat as a fuel, you can use up a significant amount of blood glucose if you walk more than two to three hours. Longer-duration activities cause your muscles to use more stored carbohydrates (muscle glycogen) and when these become depleted, you will have

---

Common Symptoms of Hypoglycemia

- Cold or clammy skin
- Dizziness or lightheadedness
- Double or blurred vision
- Elevated pulse rate (beyond exercise-induced increases)
- Headache
- Inability to do basic math
- Insomnia
- Irritability
- Mental confusion
- Nausea
- Nightmares
- Poor physical coordination
- Rapid-onset fatigue (sudden, unusual, or unexpected tiredness)
- Shakiness in your hands
- Sweating
- Tingling of hands or tongue
- Visual spots
- Weakness

---

an increased risk of developing low blood sugar, although the chances are still minimal unless you take supplemental insulin. During high-intensity, prolonged aerobic activities such as running, your body relies exclusively on carbohydrates, depleting muscle glycogen and much of the glucose in your bloodstream if you exercise for longer than two hours.

If you're controlling your diabetes with diet and exercise alone, your risk of developing low blood glucose during exercise is minimal. If your blood sugar drops during extended activities, eat an extra 4 to 15 grams of carbohydrates during or within thirty minutes of completing any glycogen-depleting exercise. Learn to recognize the symptoms of a low during or after an activity so that you can treat it.

If you take diabetic medications that increase the secretion of insulin, such as Amaryl or Glucotrol, or if you take insulin, you have a greater risk of exercise-induced lows. To prevent them, you may have to lower your insulin doses before and possibly after long exercise sessions. To participate in regular exercise training, consult with your health care provider about possibly reducing your doses of oral medications or insulin to prevent low blood sugar, particularly if you begin to experience lows related to your activities. Alternatively, you may be able to gauge how to lower preexercise insulin doses or increase carbohydrate intake by determining the glycemic effects of the activity and by using guidelines given in Dr. Sheri's book, *Diabetic Athlete's Handbook*.

Certain situations can increase the likelihood of experiencing low blood sugar, including drinking more than a couple of alcoholic drinks in the previous twelve hours, emotional stress or depression, a hypoglycemic episode in the past twenty-four to forty-eight hours, recent vigorous or prolonged exercise, a rapid drop in blood sugar (from any starting blood glucose level and for any reason), and reduced food intake. Be on the alert during exercise if any of these conditions apply to you.

Most people don't feel nearly as bad when their blood sugar is a little (or even a lot) high compared to too low, and you may feel tempted to run on the high side to prevent the lows. However, it's much better for your long-term health to try to keep your blood sugar normal and try to prevent lows.

The best treatments for hypoglycemia

Treat low blood sugar immediately with small amounts (4 to 15 grams) of high-GI carbohydrates, wait five to ten minutes for them to take effect, and then recheck your glucose levels or monitor your

---

Good Sources of Carbohydrate for Hypoglycemia Treatment

Any carbohydrates you consume during and after exercise to prevent or treat hypoglycemia should have a higher glycemic value for rapid absorption. Try consuming any of the following:

- Two to three glucose tablets (8 to 12 grams of carbohydrate) or part or all of a single glucose gel or liquid container (up to 15 grams)
- One to two pieces of hard or sugary candy (but not chocolate)
- Four ounces of regular soda
- Eight ounces of juice diluted with half water (to speed absorption)
- Eight ounces of a sports drink (6 to 9 grams of carbohydrate)
- Eight ounces of skim milk
- Two to three graham crackers or six saltines

---

symptoms. Consume the same amount of carbohydrate again only if your hypoglycemic symptoms have not begun to resolve. Avoid eating too much or you will likely end up with elevated glucose levels later on.

Glucose tablets, gels, or liquids have a couple of benefits for treating lows because glucose is the sugar that is normally in the blood and it gets there most rapidly. They also come in measured amounts—usually 4 grams of glucose per tablet or 15 grams per gel or liquid container, which makes it very easy to consume a specific number of grams of carbohydrates. With trial and error, you can determine how much each 4 gram tablet or 15 gram gel or liquid is likely to raise your blood glucose level. Never treat hypoglycemia with chocolate, doughnuts, or other high-fat sugary foods, or with low-GI carbohydrates (such as legumes), though, as they are not absorbed rapidly enough to treat lows quickly.

The best treatment will vary with the circumstances. If you're only slightly low, you may need just a tablet or two, or a small amount of glucose liquid or gel. If you're low and likely to keep dropping from whatever insulin or medication you have on board, then you may benefit by taking in some food or a drink that takes longer to digest, such as a food with fat or protein in it as well as carbohydrates like peanut butter crackers or Balance Bars. Milk is a good treatment option since it contains 7 to 8 grams of protein, along with some fat depending on what type you're drinking. Skim milk works pretty well, but at least one study showed that for prevention of lows following exercise, whole milk is much more effective than skim or even sports drinks (likely because of the milk fat).

What is hypoglycemia unawareness?

Most people who have had diabetes for longer than ten years have a blunted release of glucose-raising hormones (e.g., glucagon and adrenaline) in response to insulin-induced hypoglycemia, which increases their risk of developing lows. Mild hypoglycemic reactions are easy to treat with carbohydrate intake, but if your blood sugar drops too low without symptoms or enough time to react and treat it, you may become unresponsive or unconscious. If you ever get bad lows without being aware of it, you may have a condition known as hypoglycemia unawareness, which may affect up to 20 percent or more of insulin users. Although it's less common in people with type 2 diabetes, if you have this type and become unaware of your lows, you have a greater likelihood of experiencing severe hypoglycemia.

Normally, when your blood sugar starts to get too low, you will experience symptoms—sweating, shaking, weakness, visual changes, and others—that are caused by the release of adrenaline and the other glucose-raising hormones. If you're unaware, though, you may have either milder or missing symptoms due to this blunted hormone release. Since low blood sugar affects your ability to think

Some Tips for Preventing Hypoglycemia

- Learn your body's reaction to specific foods, activities, and stress by frequently monitoring your blood sugar to establish patterns and trends.
- Test your blood sugar more frequently whenever you're doing new activities, traveling, or deviating from your usual routine.
- If you dose with rapid-acting insulin for food intake, learn how much insulin you need for a certain intake of carbohydrate so that you don't take too much.
- Remember that it takes at least two hours for most rapid-acting insulins to clear your bloodstream; if giving additional insulin for a high within that time period, wait a while for it to exert its full effects before deciding how much more to take.
- Never skip meals or food for which you have already taken insulin or oral medications.
- If you're not sure exactly when you'll eat (as in a restaurant), don't take all of your insulin before the food arrives; rather, wait until you have it in front of you.
- Follow your blood sugar for several hours after exercise to catch and prevent postexercise delayed-onset hypoglycemia.
- Eat a carbohydrate snack (at least 15 grams) within an hour after doing strenuous or prolonged exercise to help restore your muscles' glycogen more rapidly, along with a little protein and fat that will stick around longer.

and reason, you may test your blood sugar when you're low and not realize that you need to eat, resist help from others, or even run away from paramedics.

If you effectively prevent all bouts of hypoglycemia during a three-week period, studies have shown that you will likely regain your awareness. If you often fail to sense your lows, you may consider using one of the continuous glucose monitoring devices now available to detect decreases in your blood glucose levels before they get to a critical point.

Should you exercise with elevated blood sugar?

Your body will likely respond normally to exercise with blood sugar levels up to 250 mg/dl (13.9 mmol/L) or higher. Although unlikely in type 2 diabetes, ketosis (a state of metabolic acidosis signaled by ketones in the urine) may develop in people with limited or no insulin in their bodies. If you're prone to developing ketones and your blood glucose is elevated, wait to exercise until you get rid of the ketones. They indicate that your body is deficient in insulin, and exercising can cause your blood sugar to rise more from the release of glucose-raising hormones. Having some insulin circulating in your bloodstream will help bring it down during the activity, though. Use your blood glucose meter to test your body's responses. Particularly after eating a meal when your body releases some insulin in response to food intake, your blood sugar is more likely to come down naturally when you exercise.

How important is fluid intake in preventing dehydration?

While we no longer recommend that you drink eight glasses of water a day, it is important to take in enough fluids to rehydrate yourself on a daily basis. In general, your body will need about one milliliter of fluid per calorie, or about one liter per thousand calories. Those fluids can come from water and drinks of all types (including milk, coffee, teas, cocoa, juice, etc.), as well as from water in the foods you eat. You don't have to drink water all day long to stay hydrated.

When your blood sugar is elevated, your body loses water through your urine. Be extra careful to drink enough water and fluids during and following any kind of exercise as it will be easier for you to get dehydrated. Exercising also causes you to lose more water through sweating, which can make you even more dehydrated. Be especially

---

Hydration Tips for Exercise

- Drink cool, plain water during and following exercise, especially during warmer weather, and take frequent breaks to have a chance to cool down, preferably out of the heat and direct sunlight.
- Drink only when you feel thirsty and don't force yourself to drink more than the amount of fluid that satisfies your thirst, or water intoxication may result.
- To know how much fluid to replace after exercise, weigh yourself before and after a prolonged activity and only replace up to the weight you have lost (1 liter of water weighs 1 kilogram, or 2.2 pounds).
- If you prefer fluids with some flavor, try flavored waters, sports drinks that have no added carbohydrates or calories (such as Champion Lyte), or Crystal Light.
- Drink regular sports drinks (containing glucose) only when you need carbohydrate to prevent or treat hypoglycemia during physical activities.

---

careful if exercising outdoors during hot weather; stop occasionally to rest (in the shade, if possible), and sip some fluid every ten to fifteen minutes to stay hydrated.

Is it possible to drink too much fluid?

You can become overhydrated if you drink too much, which can be as bad getting dehydrated, so don't force yourself to drink if you're not feeling thirsty. Consuming excess fluids can dilute the sodium content of your blood, causing a condition known as hyponatremia, or water intoxication, which can increase your risk for seizures, coma, and even death. Start drinking only when you actually feel thirsty or notice yourself sweating, and replace only the water you have lost (which can be determined by body weight losses).

After exercise, continue to use thirst as your guide, rehydrating with water or other calorie-free fluids. If you have consumed a lot of fluid during an activity, wait until you start to urinate before you drink any more. As for electrolytes like sodium, potassium, and chloride, you will not need to worry about replacing them during a workout unless you're exercising outdoors in hot weather for more than two hours at a time, and then replace them naturally with the foods you eat rather than taking supplements. Only use sports drinks if you need the extra carbohydrate during exercise, and don't drink more than you need to keep your blood glucose levels stable.

CARMEN DVORAK
A diabetes educator—and patient—who understands

In Chapter 1, we introduced you to Gloria Rodriguez, living well with type 2 diabetes, and you also learned about Lorena Drago, a registered dietitian and a certified diabetes educator (CDE). Now we would like to introduce a Latina who not only specializes in teaching others about diabetes but has diabetes herself: Carmen Dvorak. She had been an educator for about two years when she was diagnosed with type 2 diabetes at the young age of thirty-nine. She remembers asking herself questions like "Why me?" and "How could this happen to me?" She had never been significantly overweight, and she had been following the same meal plan as her patients since becoming an educator, as well as engaging in a regular exercise routine three days a week at her gym and walking on weekends. As a result, she lost thirteen pounds.

Carmen recalls her feelings at the time: "My mother had been diagnosed with diabetes the year before, but no one else in my family had it. After my diagnosis, I continued taking care of myself, but I was upset. One day I thought that even though diabetes is a very bad disease, one that I did not choose or want, I could at least decide for myself how I want to control it." Her diet was already good, but she rededicated herself to it. "Before I was following a meal plan that I recommend to my patients because it's healthy for everybody, but now I have to do it because

I have diabetes and want to live to be eighty years old at least and to prevent diabetes complications."

Six years into having diabetes, she is controlling it with a healthy meal plan and exercise and no medications. Her meals are balanced and consist of carbohydrates, protein, and vegetables. She admits, "I think about food all the time, but it helps me plan better and prepare a healthy meal for my family and myself." Before becoming a diabetes educator, she was not as disciplined with her meals. She thought she was eating well when she ordered chicken nuggets for her son and a fried chicken sandwich for herself as a meal, but she knows now that she was wrong. "At the beginning it just seemed like too much work to prepare a healthy meal, but in reality it's not," she says now.

As for her exercise, for the past six years Carmen has tried different types. "I get bored of doing the same type of exercise," she says. "The longest I stayed with any one was about two years. I gave up the gym after three years because I got tired of getting up at 5:00 A.M. to go there. I do exercise videos like Tai Bo or yoga some days, and on weekends I just dance salsa or merengue. I do walking while I watch TV, sometimes even just pretending that I'm on a treadmill so that I can jog. My husband and children thought that I was *loca* when they saw me in front of the TV doing exercise, but they got used to it. My family thought I was really crazy when I joined a women's soccer league at the age of forty-four. No age or disease will stop me from doing what I like and enjoy!"

As an educator who has to deal with other people's diabetes in addition to her own, she realizes how important it is to control blood sugar. She tests her sugar regularly, which helps her keep it under control. Carmen thinks that using a log book to record the results (and not just relying on the meter's memory) is important to see ranges and patterns. "I know that by controlling my sugar, I'm killing four birds with one rock," she says. "By controlling my diabetes effectively, I keep my sugar in control, but also my blood pressure and cholesterol, and I even maintain my weight."

Luckily, she is free of complications so far, but she has learned how certain things affect her control in the short term. For instance, when she is stressed, she finds that her blood sugar goes high about one hour after eating, even if she only had a small snack with about 15 grams of carbohydrate. She relates what she feels when that happens: "I feel my eyes burning and have numbness or tingling of my head and sometimes my feet too. When this happens, I try to relax by doing deep breathing exercises, drink more water, and check my sugar more frequently. If my sugar is still high before my next meal, I eat no more than 20 to 30 grams of carbohydrate and focus on eating more vegetables instead."

As a member of the Latino community, Carmen sees the barriers that exist there. She thinks the biggest hurdles are a lack of knowledge about diabetes and its possible complications and denial of its effects. "They think that because they don't feel sick or nothing hurts, they don't have diabetes or it's not that bad," she remarks. "Being a diabetes educator has definitely helped me to take control of my diabetes. Patients with access to diabetes education control their sugar better, and it helps them to prevent or delay the onset of diabetic health complications. Even a little bit of education is better than none." Her main personal barrier to good control is the "diabetes police," or relatives and friends that are always watching what she eats. On the flip side, others always offer her food and tell her to eat more since she doesn't have to worry about her weight. "I hate to be telling everybody—even people I don't know—that I have diabetes, but I do so that they stop pushing food on me!"

When asked her secrets for living long and well with diabetes (including what she is doing for herself and recommends to her patients), Carmen gave the following list: (1) ask your doctor for diabetes education as soon as he or she tells you that you have diabetes or "a little sugar" in your blood; (2) check your blood sugar regularly; (3) eat healthy, balanced meals, including breakfast, lunch, dinner, and a snack, and never go more than five hours without eating during the day; (4) exercise regularly—at least three days a week for thirty minutes—and try to park away from the entrance door to the mall or grocery store so that you can get extra steps that way or walk in front of the TV while watching your favorite programs; and (5) take your medication as prescribed by your doctor, but make sure to inform him if you have side effects, if your sugar goes too low, or if it does not come down. She also advises that you don't stop taking any medication without informing your doctor.

Exercising with diabetic or other health limitations: ¡No problema!

What is your biggest excuse for not being more physically active? The purpose of this section is to persuade you to give up your health-related excuses, even if you suffer from high blood pressure, loss of feeling in your feet, or arthritic knees or hips. Older individuals with chronic health problems respond just as well to exercise training as younger folks, so suboptimal health no longer needs to be your reason for inactivity (even though 85 percent of people over sixty-five have a health problem that they often view as a deterrent). Although most everyone can exercise safely and effectively, diabetes does carry some additional risks. To stay safe and get the most out of your activities, follow the exercise guidelines published by the American Diabetes Association and respect your limitations while staying as physically active as possible.

How to exercise safely with heart disease

If you have diabetes or prediabetes, you may also already have the beginnings of cardiovascular disease, which can cause heart attack, stroke, ischemia (reduced blood flow to your heart), or reduced leg blood flow, but none of these should prevent you from exercising. Diabetic people in supervised cardiac rehabilitation exercise programs engage in various forms of exercise, and you may choose to join such a program if you know you have cardiovascular disease, or you may prefer to exercise on your own or with others. Regular exercise helps improve blood flow through your body and reduce the severity of cardiovascular changes you may already be experiencing.

If you experience angina (chest pain) due to reduced blood flow to your heart muscle (a condition known as ischemia) during an aerobic activity like walking, you will actually be less likely to have the same problem during resistance workouts. Studies have shown that lifting a heavy weight ten to twelve times may increase your blood pressure more than aerobic exercise does, but it doesn't raise your heart rate as much. The higher blood pressure causes your heart muscle to get more blood during this type of workout than it does during aerobic activities. If you have some coronary artery blockage from plaque buildup, moderate weight training may be a safer activity for you than most higher-intensity aerobic ones, and resistance training is recommended nowadays for almost everyone to increase strength and preserve muscle mass.

If you prefer walking but experience angina with exertion, simply keep your heart rate about ten beats per minute lower than the point at which you start to experience pain or tightness in your chest during the activity: For example, reach no higher than 120 beats per minute if you have symptoms of ischemia at a heart rate of 130. You also need to realize that a heart attack may have symptoms other than pain localized in your chest, such as pain or discomfort that radiates down one arm or shoulder or your neck or that feels like bad heartburn. If you experience unusual pain or other symptoms during or following exercise, get checked out by your doctor as soon as possible. If you experience a sudden, unexplained change in your ability to exercise (such as extreme fatigue that comes on quickly), without any other symptoms, immediately stop exercising and consult with your physician as soon as you can to rule out silent ischemia (a symptomless reduction in heart blood flow) as well.

Exercising slightly increases your risk of having a cardiovascular event during the activity, but regular exercise actually lowers your chances. Nonetheless, it's in your best interest to know the usual warning symptoms of heart attack or stroke. Don't delay in seeking immediate medical attention, preferably through activating EMS

Heart Attack Warning Signs

- Chest discomfort: in the center of the chest that lasts or is intermittent. It sometimes feels like bad indigestion, or it can feel like uncomfortable pressure, squeezing, fullness, or acute and stabbing pain.
- Discomfort elsewhere: pain or discomfort radiating down one or both arms, the back, neck, jaw, or stomach. This symptom is referred pain, which is actually originating in your heart due to lack of proper oxygen.
- Shortness of breath, particularly when it is unusual or unexpected. It can occur with or without chest discomfort.
- Other symptoms: sudden sweating, nausea and vomiting, lightheadedness, or undue, unexplained fatigue.

---

by calling 911, if you are experiencing any of them. Treatment in the first few minutes is critical for surviving a major cardiac event with a minimum of lasting problems.

Should leg pain keep you from exercising?

Peripheral artery disease (PAD), a form of cardiovascular disease, is a common circulatory problem that limits blood flow to the legs and arms. Plaque can form in any artery, not just the ones feeding the heart and brain, and PAD usually occurs in peripheral arteries in the legs. Pain in your lower legs while standing or walking is a common symptom, but PAD can also be a sign that you have widespread plaque formation in other arteries around your body. If plaque formations in your leg arteries rupture, you can experience a blockage that limits or cuts off blood supply to the lower legs, resulting in pain, changes in skin color, sores or ulcers, difficult walking, and even gangrene.

If you experience symptoms in your legs during or after physical activity and you have not yet been diagnosed with PAD, confer with your physician to get a definite diagnosis before proceeding with your exercise program. PAD can be diagnosed by measuring the blood pressure in your leg and comparing it to the blood pressure in your arm. If they're unequal, you may have blockage in your lower limbs that is raising the pressure there. However, you can get your PAD under control and maintain your normal activities. In fact, walking or other daily exercise is a key to maintaining optimal circulation in your legs, along with a healthy diet and smoking cessation. You may have to choose activities that do not result in pain, such as seated exercises, water workouts, upper body resistance training, or stationary cycling. In addition, certain prescribed medications that lower your blood pressure can dilate your leg arteries, and surgery can improve blood flow to your legs by bypassing blockages.

Which activities are better if you have high blood pressure?

Regular aerobic exercise lessens the potential impact of most other cardiovascular risk factors, including elevated blood lipids (cholesterol and other blood fats), insulin resistance, obesity, and hypertension. Hypertension is associated with high levels of insulin in your body, which are common with insulin resistance. The good news is that regular physical activity can result in lower blood pressure and reduced circulating levels of insulin, making it very beneficial to your health.

If you have elevated blood pressure, you may need to avoid high-intensity or heavy resistance exercises that can cause your blood pressure to rise dangerously high and precipitate a stroke or heart attack. Limit your involvement in heavy weight training; near-maximal exercise of any type; activities that require intense, sustained contractions of the upper body, such as waterskiing or windsurfing; or any exercise that involves holding your breath.

Being active with peripheral neuropathy and lower limb ulcers

Loss of sensation or pain in your feet or hands is called peripheral neuropathy, and if you have it, your risk of damaging your feet or lower limbs during exercise increases greatly since it can blunt your ability to sense what is going on with them. If you don't get the usual symptoms of pain or discomfort resulting from impact on your feet or friction and pressure from footwear, it is much easier to develop a blister or sore on your foot without being aware of it. In some cases, a simple blister can progress to a full-blown infected abscess or ulcer and ultimately result in a lower-limb amputation, if not detected and treated in time.

If you have lost sensation in your feet, the American Diabetes Association recommends that you use shoes with silica gel or air midsoles (the middle section of the shoe that provides the most stability and shock absorption), along with polyester or cotton-polyester socks, to prevent blisters and keep your feet dry during physical activities. Pure cotton socks are not recommended because they tend to get wet, which may promote damage to your feet. You (or someone else) will need to check your feet daily for signs of trauma and treat them aggressively to prevent any worsening of any problems that arise.

If you have lost feeling in your feet or have ulcerated skin, it may also be a good idea to switch to activities such as swimming or stationary cycling that minimize the trauma to your lower extremities and the ulcerated area. Good exercises include all aquatic activities (swimming, pool walking, and water aerobics), upper-body exercises (rowing, arm crank ergometers), chair exercises, stationary cycling, yoga, and abdominal work. These activities also improve your body tone, balance, and awareness of your lower extremities.

Although regular exercise does not reverse peripheral neuropathy, it can slow its progression and prevent further loss of fitness from occurring due to inactivity. It may also improve circulation in your lower legs and feet and help prevent ulcers. Research has recently shown that even deconditioned individuals with diabetic neuropathies respond well to combined resistance and interval exercise training. If your peripheral nerve damage causes dull, shooting, or throbbing pain in your extremities after you go for a walk or engage in other weight-bearing activities, though, remember to limit that activity in the future and switch to others that don't cause you lasting pain or discomfort. If the pain is constant, you may need to seek treatment for painful diabetic neuropathy or be tested for PAD.

What are the exercise concerns with central nerve damage?

If you have damage to your central nervous system (autonomic neuropathy), you're more likely to experience silent ischemia, which could result in a "silent" or undetected heart attack. Your chances of dying suddenly during exercise from such an event are high once your heart has become unresponsive to nerve impulses, particularly if you have some level of underlying heart disease. If severe, this complication may also make it harder for you to change your body position (e.g., going from sitting to standing or from lying to sitting) without experiencing orthostatic hypotension (a drop in blood pressure) that can cause lightheadedness or fainting. You're also more likely to overheat and get dehydrated. If it has also affected your ability to digest and absorb foods (known as gastroparesis), any carbohydrate you eat to treat a low blood glucose reaction during exercise might be more slowly absorbed, and your hypoglycemia might become more severe as a result. Finally, this complication may cause you to have an elevated heart rate at rest (e.g., 100 beats per minute or higher instead of the normal 72), and it can keep your heart from beating as fast as it should once you start to exercise.

If you have been diagnosed with autonomic nerve damage, take a conservative approach to exercise. Try to avoid rapid changes in movement that may result in fainting and take ten minutes or more to warm up and cool down, particularly when you're doing strenuous activities. Drink extra fluid during exercise and avoid being continuously active for long periods during hot weather. Avoid eating a large meal before exercise as it could result in delayed emptying of food from your stomach; eat small portions beforehand. To treat a low, take glucose tablets before your blood glucose levels reach 100 mg/dl to prevent severe hyperglycemia. Finally, use a subjective rating (e.g., "somewhat hard") to monitor the difficulty level of your workout in place of just measuring your exertion by heart rate as it may no longer rise as much as normal due to nerve damage.

Exercise precautions with diabetic eye disease

People with diabetes often develop eye complications, including cataracts and retinopathy. Cataracts can obscure your vision and make participation in certain activities (e.g., outdoor cycling) more dangerous, but they're not usually a complete barrier to exercise. More severe forms of eye disease like proliferative diabetic retinopathy, however, can cause your eyes to form weak, abnormal blood vessels in the back of the eye (the retina) that can break, tear, or bleed into the vitreous fluid in the center of your eye, filling it with blood that can obscure vision temporarily or permanently. If you have severe or unstable eye disease, you will need to make greater changes to your exercise regimen to prevent bleeding into your eye.

Precautions for Exercising with Diabetes and Its Complications

- Have a blood glucose meter accessible to check your blood glucose level before, possibly during, and/or after exercise, or if you have any symptoms of low sugar.
- Immediately treat low blood glucose during or following exercise with easily absorbed carbohydrates like glucose tablets or regular soft drinks.
- Inform your exercise partner(s) about your diabetes, and show them how to administer glucose or another carbohydrate to you should you need assistance in treating a low.
- Stay properly hydrated with frequent sips of cool water.
- Consult with your physician prior to exercising with any of the following conditions:
  - Proliferative retinopathy or current retinal hemorrhage
  - Neuropathy (nerve damage), either peripheral or autonomic
  - Foot injuries (including ulcers)
  - High blood pressure
  - Serious illness or infection
- Seek immediate medical attention for chest pain or any pain or discomfort that radiates down your arm, jaw, or neck.
- If you have hypertension, avoid activities that cause large increases in your blood pressure, such as heavy resistance work, head-down exercises, and anything that forces you to hold your breath.
- Wear proper footwear, and check your feet daily for signs of trauma such as blisters, redness, or other irritation.
- Stop exercising immediately if you experience bleeding into your eyes caused by active proliferative retinopathy.
- Wear a diabetes medic alert bracelet or necklace with your physician's name and contact information on it.

While exercise doesn't accelerate the proliferative process, you will need to take certain precautions to prevent intra-ocular hemorrhages or retinal tears. If your eye disease is only mild or moderate, with no active bleeds, avoid activities that dramatically increase the blood pressure inside your eyes, such as heavy weight lifting or activities with your head lower than your heart. If you have moderate to severe diabetic eye disease, do not engage in activities that involve jumping, jarring, or breath holding. They increase the pressure inside your eyes and can cause more bleeding and increase your risk of retinal tears or retinal detachment. Activities best avoided include boxing, competitive contact sports (such as basketball and football), jogging, high-impact aerobics, most racquet sports, and heavy weight lifting. If you have an active retinal hemorrhage or notice sudden, dramatic changes in your sight, stop any activity you are doing immediately and check with your eye doctor for further guidance.

Is exercise possible with diabetic kidney disease?

Exercise does not appear to worsen diabetes-related kidney problems (nephropathy). Intense or prolonged exercise is not recommended if you have full-blown kidney disease, however, because while kidney damage will not potentially result from the activity, your physical capacity for exercise is likely to be limited. Light to moderate exercise is well tolerated, though, and patients requiring dialysis can exercise regularly—even during dialysis treatments—without ill effects. If you are undergoing dialysis, only avoid exercising if the levels of certain substances in your blood (hematocrit or total red blood cell count, calcium, or potassium) become unbalanced as a result of the treatments or if you experience extreme fatigue immediately following a dialysis session. People who have undergone kidney transplants can safely exercise six to eight weeks after surgery, once they are stable and free of signs of rejection of the new kidney.

You may not be aware that exercise can increase the urinary excretion of protein or microalbumin, both of which are potential indicators of kidney problems. For your peace of mind and to prevent false conclusions, abstain from exercising on a day that you are collecting your urine for either of these tests so that your results will not be erroneously skewed and misinterpreted as evidence of kidney damage or disease progression.

Dealing with arthritis and other joint problems

Being overweight increases your risk for arthritis in the hips, knees, and ankles, which may limit your ability to exercise. Research has clearly shown that exercise is an effective means of managing arthritis, though, even the more severe rheumatoid type. Start with basic range of motion exercises (including stretching) to increase your joint mobility, and then move on to specific resistance work that strengthens the muscles surrounding affected joints. This will also help you maintain your leg strength, which is critical to basic movements like getting up out of a chair, climbing stairs, and walking. If you have arthritic knees or hips, walking may be uncomfortable or painful. Your best option is to try non–weight bearing activities, such as walking in a pool (with or without a flotation belt around your waist), aqua aerobics, lap swimming, recumbent stationary cycling, upper-body exercises, seated aerobic workouts, and resistance activities. It helps to vary your activities so that you're stressing your joints differently each day. For best results, warm up and cool down properly to ease your joint transition into and out of each workout.

Diabetes increases your risk of experiencing joint-related injuries and overuse problems like tendonitis, so it may be prudent to choose a more moderate exercise like walking rather than jogging or running to reduce the potential for joint trauma. Diabetic frozen shoulder, trigger finger, and other acute joint problems can also come on with no warning and for no apparent reason, even if you exercise regularly and moderately. The best defense against injuries is good blood glucose control as well as flexibility exercise.

After exercising, you may want to apply ice to your joints (particularly knees) for fifteen to twenty minutes to reduce swelling and help prevent soreness. In addition, consider taking nonsteroidal, anti-inflammatory medications like aspirin or ibuprofen to lessen any residual discomfort.

Having a disability that leaves you with limited mobility or in a wheelchair does not mean that you can't be regularly active. Working just your upper body can increase your mobility as you gain enhanced upper-body strength, endurance, and flexibility. Any type of activity can also give you most of exercise's health benefits, even if you do it sitting in a chair or wheelchair.

Dealing with injuries or muscle soreness due to exercise

Whenever you engage in a new exercise, expect some soreness or stiffness to follow in the next day or two. Stretch out your tight muscles and joints after workouts. If you feel sore the day after exercise, try some gentle warm-up and cool-down exercises. If your mobility is limited, you are likely experiencing delayed-onset muscle soreness (DOMS). Although unpleasant, DOMS requires no special treatment other than time and often feels better if you do light exercise, take a hot bath or get in a hot tub, stretch, or gently massage the affected muscles. Luckily your body responds by building stress proteins into the repaired muscles, making it very hard to reach that same level of soreness in the same muscles for six to eight weeks afterward, even if you overdo it again.

Having intense or lasting pain after exercise is not normal or expected. If you do get injured (which you'll know from the sharp, localized pain you'll feel during or immediately after training), treat it with standard RICE techniques—rest, ice, compression, and elevation. As soon as the injury improves, ease slowly back into your exercise routine. Be sure to have the injury checked out by a physician if it doesn't start to get better within a week.

You can get an acute injury by using improper exercise techniques or through carelessness (e.g., dropping a dumbbell on your foot). More likely, though, if you develop an injury, it will be the result of excessive training that results from doing too much too soon. This type of injury is nagging and persistently uncomfortable. By definition, an overuse injury is caused by excessive use of a particular joint. These injuries are more common when you have diabetes because elevated blood sugars can affect the health of your joints. Regardless of the cause, treat them with RICE techniques, combined with anti-inflammatory medications like ibuprofen (Advil or Nuprin) or naproxen sodium (found in Aleve).

If you properly care for your injuries, they should start to get better within 7 days. If not, or if you have a single point of intense pain, you should see a physician (preferably a podiatrist who has expertise in foot, ankle, and lower leg problems as well as diabetes) who can pinpoint the cause of your discomfort with an X-ray, bone scan, or MRI. You may need physical therapy or rehabilitation for persistent problems.

Avoid going back to your normal activities until your symptoms have gone away. Cross training is one way to deal with injuries without losing all of your conditioning while waiting for the injury to heal. If you have lower leg pain, you can still work out your upper body doing other activities and vice versa. Try to alternate weight-bearing activities like walking with non–weight bearing ones (e.g., swimming and stationary cycling) to avoid injuring another part of your body while waiting for an injury to heal. To prevent the recurrence of an injury once you can resume your normal

General Tips for Safe and Effective Exercise

- Never bounce during stretches; doing so can cause injuries.
- If you haven't exercised in a while, start out slowly and progress cautiously.
- Warm up with stretches and easy aerobic work before you exercise more vigorously.
- Choose an exercise that suits your condition; for example, swimming might be better for those who find walking difficult.
- Find an exercise partner to help you stay motivated.
- Set goals to keep your interest up; for instance, if you walk for exercise, get a pedometer and set a goal of adding in 2,000 more steps each day.
- Reward yourself when you reach goals (but preferably not with food).
- Vary your exercise program occasionally or try out new activities to stay motivated. Variety also emphasizes different muscle groups and increases your overall fitness.
- Cross train to reduce the risk of injury by varying muscle usage.
- Wear appropriate shoes and socks, and check your feet after you exercise.
- When you start a new exercise, check your blood glucose levels before, during (if more than an hour), and after your workout.
- Don't forget to warm up and cool down for best results.

activities, work on strengthening the muscles around the affected area. Following a shoulder joint injury, for example, focus on doing resistance work using all sections of the deltoid muscle, as well as biceps, triceps, pectorals, and upper back and neck muscles, to strengthen the muscles around that area of your body.

CHAPTER 6: *En pocas palabras*

Anyone can exercise safely and effectively, even with diabetes-related health complications or arthritis. If you have any concerns, consider having a checkup before starting an exercise program. It is also important to learn how to prevent low or high blood sugar during and following exercise, along with dehydration. Even if you have heart disease, leg pain, nerve damage, eye problems, kidney damage, arthritis, or other problems, you can find a way to be more physically active. You simply need to learn how to respect your body's limitations and work around them.

CHAPTER 7

Treating Your Diabetes Right: Monitoring and Medications

Multiple research studies have shown that achieving good diabetes control is more challenging for Latinos than it is for others in the United States. Many Latinos have low incomes compared to whites and other non-Latino minorities, limited access to health care, and no health insurance. Typically, diabetic Latinos have A1c tests (indicating overall blood glucose control over the previous two to three months) that are 0.5 percent higher than non-Hispanic whites and other ethnic groups. Regardless of the causes of such disparities, what can you do to combat these problems? We'll address these issues in this chapter, along with discussing the importance of home blood glucose monitoring and making the best use of the wide variety of diabetic medications available today.

Why is using a blood glucose meter so important?

One characteristic of people living successfully with any type of diabetes is that they use their blood glucose meters religiously. You can use frequent testing to detect patterns and to learn your body's unique response to different things—foods, activities, medications, emotional and physical stress, and more—so that you can adjust your medications or insulin to work for you as effectively as possible to control your blood glucose and prevent future health complications.

Testing your blood sugar at different times—rather than just first thing in the morning or before meals—can often reveal trends with your blood glucose levels that you might not notice otherwise. For example, you may wake up every day and test, and your blood sugar is fairly consistent. But do you know what it is doing the rest of the day? What effect does eating beans and rice have on it compared with chicken or fish? If you don't immediately know the answer to these questions, then you should consider occasionally testing at alternate times, even if you don't increase the number of times a day that you test to save money on strips for your meter.

Postmeal glucose excursions (i.e., how much your blood sugar goes up in the two hours after a meal) may be just as important in causing diabetic complications as overall glucose control—maybe even more so. We do know that controlling such spikes may be the key to preventing microvascular complications like diabetic retinopathy. Testing not only before meals, but also one hour and two hours afterward can let you know how your various meals are affecting your blood glucose levels and how much variability in your glucose levels you are experiencing. Regardless of which type of diabetes you have, your blood sugar typically reaches a peak seventy-two minutes after you start eating (give or take twenty-three minutes), and both the American Diabetes Association and the American Association of Clinical Endocrinologists recommend checking blood glucose levels two hours after your first bite of a meal. For better control of your diabetes, then, consider varying your blood glucose testing instead of always testing at the same time each day.

What is your glycated hemoglobin goal?

If you have diabetes, you should routinely get your glycated hemoglobin (A1c) tested every three to six months. As discussed in Chapter 1, this blood test tells you how much glucose is bound onto a certain part of the hemoglobin molecules in your red blood cells. As your blood sugar runs higher, a greater percentage of them will have glucose "stuck" on them for the remainder of the red blood cell's life, which is usually two to three months. So, the value gives you an idea how your blood sugar has been averaging during the past several months, particularly the previous four weeks. The current recommendations are for everyone to have a value of 7 percent or less. Some groups recommend a goal of less than 6.5 percent, and normal values usually fall in the range of 4.0 of 6.0 percent. The closer you are to normal, the better for your health.

Estimated average glucose (eAG):
An easier way to interpret your A1c

Recently there has been a push to convert the A1c value into an equivalent glucose reading to make it more meaningful when you see it. This new value, the eAG, or estimated average glucose, immediately tells you what your glucose has been in the values you are used to seeing—either mg/dl (in the United States) or millimolar (mmol/L, in other countries). (For more information, see Table 7.1.) The relationship between A1c and eAG follows this formula:

28.7 x A1c - 46.7 = eAG in mg/dl
(For values in mmol/L, divide the number you get by 18.)

You can alternately use an online tool that converts your A1c for you, accessible here: professional.diabetes.org/glucosecalculator .aspx.

The only thing this value can't tell you is how high your blood glucose spikes after meals, which may contribute to the development of diabetic complications. If your eAG (or equivalent A1c) reading is higher than the average you have on your blood glucose meter, then you may be having high postmeal sugars (when you didn't test) that you need to control better to avoid getting diabetes-related complications.

Table 7.1: Estimated Average Glucose (eAG) Based on Equivalent A1c Values

A1c	eAG: mg/dl	(mmol/L)
5%	97	(5.4)
5.5%	112	(6.2)
6%	126	(7.0)
6.5%	140	(7.8)
7%	154	(8.6)
7.5%	169	(9.4)
8%	183	(10.1)
8.5%	197	(10.9)
9%	212	(11.8)
9.5%	226	(12.6)
10%	240	(13.4)
10.5%	255	(14.1)
11%	269	(14.9)
11.5%	283	(15.7)
12%	298	(16.5)
13%	326	(18.1)
14%	365	(20.3)

Is blood glucose all you have to worry about?

If you have diabetes—especially when it is not well controlled—you may also have elevated blood fat levels (cholesterol and triglycerides). See Table 7.2 for recommended levels. Doctors often prescribe cholesterol-lowering medications, the most popular being the statins (e.g., Lipitor, Mevacor, Pravachol, Crestor, and Zocor). Not only do these medications lower levels of harmful cholesterol (LDL cholesterol), but they also appear to help protect your cardiovascular health by preventing blood clots (a common precipitator of heart attack and stroke), improving blood flow (endothelial function), and lowering inflammation (a primary contributor to insulin resistance).

Taking medications is not the only way to lower blood cholesterol levels, though. Getting more exercise, improving your diet, controlling your blood sugar, losing some body weight, and eating plenty of fiber all help reduce cholesterol, often just as effectively as taking additional medications—without the cost or the side effects. Regardless of how you achieve your goals, the overall goal of all of these measurements is, of course, to maintain your health in an optimal range throughout your life. Strive to maintain your blood glucose levels, blood fats, and blood pressure in a normal range (or as near to normal as you can get) at all times. But keep your control in perspective and don't obsess over it because this can have the opposite effect on your health.

Using pills to control your diabetes

For people with type 2 diabetes, taking oral diabetic medications may be an important step in controlling blood sugar, and there are many medications to choose from, discussed in the sections that follow (and listed in Table 7.3). Several older classes of oral medications are still used, along with metformin (sold as Glucophage),

Table 7.2: Target Goals for Blood Glucose, Cholesterol, and Blood Pressure

	Fasting (overnight)	Throughout the Day
Blood glucose (mg/dl)	70-120 (before meals) (3.9-6.7 mmol/L)	<180 (2 hours after meals) (10.0 mmol/L)
Glycated hemoglobin (A1c) (%)	<7.0 (American Diabetes Association goal)	<6.5 (American Association of Clinical Endocrinologists)
Estimated average glucose (eAG) (mg/dl)	<154 (8.6 mmol/L)	<140 (7.8 mmol/L)
Total Cholesterol (mg/dl)	<200	<180 (even better)
HDL-cholesterol (mg/dl)	>40 for males, >50 for females	>60 (optimal for everyone)
LDL-cholesterol (mg/dl)	<100 (for diabetes)	<70 (for higher heart disease risk)
Triglycerides (mg/dl)	<150	
Blood pressure (mm Hg)	<120/<80	Never over 130/85

which targets the liver to reduce its blood glucose production overnight and after meals, and increases insulin action around the body. If your fasting glucose levels are typically high, this drug is usually prescribed. Sulfonylureas like Amaryl and Glyburide help stimulate your pancreas to make more insulin (if it can). Both Actos and Avandia, drugs in the thiazolidinedione (TZD) class, work by sensitizing fat and muscle cells to insulin. Combination drugs that incorporate two of these classes of drugs in one pill are catching on, since multiple drugs are often prescribed to control type 2 diabetes. For instance, Glucovance and Metaglip combine a sulfonylurea and

Table 7.3: Oral and Other Diabetic Medications

Class of Drug	Examples (Brand Name)	Mechanism of Action(s)
Sulfonylureas	Amaryl, DiaBeta, Diabinese, Glynase, Glucotrol, Micronase, Glyburide, Orinase	Promote insulin secretion from the beta cells of the pancreas; some may increase insulin sensitivity
Biguanides	Glucophage (metformin), Glucophage XR, Riomet, Glumetza	Decrease liver glucose output; increase liver and muscle insulin sensitivity; no direct effect on beta cells
Thiazolidinediones "Glitazones"	Avandia, Actos	Increase insulin sensitivity of peripheral tissues, such as muscle
DPP-4 Inhibitors	Januvia, Galvus	Work by inhibiting DPP-4, an enzyme that breaks down glucagon-like peptide-1 (GLP-1); delayed GLP-1 degradation extends the action of insulin while suppressing glucagon release
Meglitinides/ Phenylalanine derivatives	Prandin, Starlix	Stimulate beta cells to increase insulin secretion, but only for a very short duration (unlike sulfonylureas)
Alpha-Glucosidase Inhibitors	Precose, Glyset	Work in intestines to slow digestion of some carbohydrates to control post-meal blood glucose peaks
Amylin	Symlin (injected)	Works in combination with insulin to control glycemic spikes for three hours after meals
Incretins and incretin mimetics	Byetta (injected)	Stimulate insulin release; inhibit the liver's release of glucose via glucagon; delay the emptying of food from the stomach

a biguanide, and Avandamet is a combination of a glitazone and a biguanide. If you have type 1 diabetes, though, most of these medications will not help control your diabetes (with the possible exception of metformin).

Sulfonylureas. The medications that have been around longest for the treatment of type 2 diabetes are the sulfonylureas (e.g., Amaryl, DiaBeta, Diabinese, Glynase, Glucotrol, and Micronase), which work by stimulating your pancreas to produce more insulin. The newer generation of sulfonylureas has fewer potential side effects than the older ones. If your pancreas eventually loses the capacity to make much insulin, no medication will be able to stimulate your beta cells to make enough to control your blood glucose levels effectively. Although your glycemic control may initially be improved by adding a sulfonylurea to a biguanide (discussed next), your blood glucose levels are likely to resume their deterioration in as little as six months after you start using the medications together. These medications are generally less expensive than the newer ones, however.

Biguanides. Metformin is the generic name of the only compound in this class with FDA approval marketed under several different trade names, such as Glucophage and Glucophage XR. Its primary advantage over sulfonylureas is that it doesn't induce hypoglycemia when taken alone. Rather, it shuts down your liver's excessive production of glucose overnight, making it excellent for treating morning hyperglycemia. It additionally improves the action of your insulin in both your liver and your muscles. As the only oral diabetic medication that promotes weight loss, it is frequently prescribed as the drug of first choice. But it only facilitates weight loss if you use Glucophage rather than an extended release form (e.g., Glucophage XR or Glumetza). Although metformin appears to be somewhat protective of the heart compared with other diabetic medications, it potentially causes mild nausea and diarrhea. Taking it with meals generally decreases these symptoms, as does using the extended release forms. If you come down with an acute illness while taking it, you may have to discontinue it until you're well, as it may cause lactic acid to build up in your circulation. It can reverse ovulatory abnormalities found in some overweight women, however, leading to a greater risk of unplanned pregnancies in premenopausal women.

Thiazolidinediones. Medications that act to increase insulin action, the thiazolidinediones (TZDs) mimic the insulin-sensitizing effects of physical activity. Two medications in this class, Avandia and Actos, are available by prescription, although Avandia has recently been investigated as possibly contributing to heart failure (both now have black box warnings on them for this reason), and both may increase the risk of bone fractures in older women. Both improve insulin sensitivity, do not cause hypoglycemia, and can be taken once daily. In addition to increasing your muscles' use of blood glucose at rest, they also increase your body's responsiveness to circulating insulin during exercise but are not likely to cause exercise-induced low blood sugar.

DPP-4 Inhibitors. A recently approved class of *medicamentos orales* for people with type 2 diabetes includes two medications, Januvia and Galvus, which work with gut hormones, natural enzymes, and the body's own insulin to control blood glucose levels. In addition to having few side effects, these medications apparently lessen the notorious effects of other oral medications (e.g., nausea). Incretin hormones, called GLP-1 and GIP, are naturally occurring substances produced in the intestines in response to food intake; they help regulate blood sugar by stimulating both the alpha and beta cells of the pancreas. Alpha cells secrete a hormone called glucagon, which mobilizes glucose when your blood sugar is low (such as overnight or during prolonged activity). The incretin response is much less effective in people with diabetes, and their pancreatic islet cells function progressively worse. These medications boost the incretin response by inhibiting DPP-4, an enzyme that breaks down incretin hormones before they have time to work effectively. Recent studies also suggest that DPP-4 inhibitors may preserve the life and function of insulin-producing beta cells as well.

Meglitinides. Other type 2 diabetic medications include the meglitinides, Prandin and Starlix, which work well if you eat sporadically. You can take a dose only when you eat to cause your pancreas to release enough insulin to cover any blood glucose spikes. If you experience sharply rising blood glucose levels shortly after eating, you will definitely benefit from using them, assuming that your beta cells still have the capacity to sufficiently increase their insulin release. They are also safe for use by pregnant women with gestational diabetes.

Alpha-glucosidase inhibitors. Another class of FDA-approved medications, alpha-glucosidase inhibitors, control your glycemic spikes by slowing the absorption of carbohydrates from your stomach after eating, if you take a dose immediately before meals. Even pregnant women with gestational diabetes can safely use either Precose or Glyset, the two approved medications in this class, to help control rising glucose levels after meals. These medications, however, are not advised if your digestion is slowed by gastroparesis (caused by autonomic nerve damage).

Combination therapies. It is important to avoid extended periods of hyperglycemia, so if you can't adequately control your blood glucose levels within the first three to six months on a medication like metformin despite increasing your dosage, your physician will likely talk to you about adding additional therapies. Even if your physician put you on only one diabetic medication to start, it's common to end up being prescribed two or more to use simultane-

---

MARIA DE LOS ANGELES MARTINEZ DE POZOS
Diabetes runs in her family

A resident of Mexico, Maria de los Angeles Martinez de Pozos has lived with type 2 diabetes for more than thirteen years. Although her brother, aunt, and cousin also have type 2, she still remembers feeling sad and angry about her own diagnosis. "At the beginning, I was really sad because having diabetes means a big change in your life," she remarks. In fact, her emotions remain her biggest barrier to effectively controlling the disease. To deal with them, she has found that doing relaxing exercises and walking for forty-five minutes a day work best. "Mental control is very important," she remarks, "as well as being positive. If you can do those things, everything will seem worth it, and your diabetes treatment will work as well as you wish."

Although she has type 2 diabetes, Maria takes two doses of NPH insulin every day, one in the morning and another in the evening. She also eats about 1,500 calories per day. She believes that discipline is the key to living long and well with diabetes, and she practices what she preaches, particularly when it comes to her diet. "I have a whole list of foods that I avoid," she says. "It includes cakes, candies, chocolates, sodas, natural or bottled juice, cheese, pasta, pork, and sausage." Instead, she focuses on eating small portions of carbohydrate foods like rice and whole wheat bread, along with chicken, vegetables, strawberries, turkey, ham, sugar-free jelly, and more. She also drinks about three liters of water every day.

Maria agrees that lacking information about diabetes and economic resources is the main barrier to good diabetes control for the people of Mexico. She says, "It is very important to read as much as possible about diabetes. This way, it will be easier for you to control it. You also learn to live with it and make diabetes a part of your life."

---

ously. When the first prescribed medication fails to adequately control your blood glucose levels, the standard medical practice is to add in another, initiating a combination therapy. Fortunately, though, newer compounds such as Byetta have recently been shown to reduce the need for additional medications once maximal doses of combination oral therapies have begun to fail. In addition, recently discovered genes that may be responsible for weight gain and type 2 diabetes will likely be the targets of the next generation of medications, and some may be able to prevent diabetes altogether. Finally, immune suppression alone or in combination with therapies promoting beta cell regrowth may enable your own pancreas to start producing adequate amounts of insulin again.

What is Symlin used for?

A synthetic form of a natural hormone called amylin, which is normally released along with insulin by your beta cells, Symlin (generic name: pramlintide), is one of the newer medications for treating diabetes. If your body makes very little or no insulin, then you are missing the natural release of this hormone, which is why Symlin is prescribed for people with type 1 diabetes or with type 2 using insulin. One drawback is that it can only be injected, not taken by mouth. Its main action is to work with insulin following meals to control the flow of glucose into your circulation coming from digested foods. Symlin use can cause severe hypoglycemia (the risk is greater in type 1s), nausea, vomiting, abdominal pain, headache, fatigue, and dizziness. People with gastroparesis should not use this medication as it can cause them to develop severe hypoglycemia. A potential benefit is that Symlin can help you lose weight, possibly due to tighter blood glucose control and early satiety. It can also reduce oxidative stress that contributes to the development of diabetic complications.

What are the effects of incretins and incretin mimetics?

A class of diabetic medications known as incretins and incretin mimetics has recently been approved for use in the treatment of type

2 diabetes. One of these compounds (exenatide) received FDA approval under the trade name Byetta, which is actually a synthetic version of a small protein derived from the venom of the Gila monster (a poisonous lizard found in the southwestern United States and Mexico). Incretins (and synthetic versions of them) are gut hormones that stimulate the initial release of insulin in response to food you eat (a response that is missing in most people with diabetes), protect your pancreatic beta cells from burnout (the main reason for the failure of other diabetic drugs), inhibit your liver's release of glucose (by blocking glucagon release), delay the emptying of food from your stomach, and promote early feelings of fullness—usually causing you to lose weight as an added benefit. Despite occasional side effects such as nausea, vomiting, transient headaches, and increased risk of hypoglycemia when used in combination with sulfonylureas, this newest class of medications replaces the natural hormones normally released by the digestive tract after meals to spur insulin release and provides another choice for diabetes treatment, particularly if your treatment with sulfonylureas or other compounds is no longer working effectively. A drawback for many potential users, though, is that it has to be injected (rather than ingested) twice a day, although a once-weekly form will likely soon be available.

Exercise precautions when using oral diabetic medications (or Symlin or Byetta)

Certain medications, including some of the oral diabetic ones, can affect your body's response to exercise, depending on how they work. These medications target one or more of the metabolic dysfunctions caused by diabetes: insulin release from the pancreatic beta cells; the liver's production of blood glucose; and insulin resistance in fat tissues, the liver, or muscles. Older-generation sulfonylureas (such as

Diabinese and Orinase) cause insulin to be released from the pancreas and reduce insulin resistance. These older medications typically have a longer duration (up to seventy-two hours) than the newer sulfonylureas, though, giving these older ones the greatest potential to cause a low blood sugar level during and possibly after exercise.

Second-generation sulfonylureas, such as Amaryl, DiaBeta, Micronase, and Glucotrol, generally don't last as long and carry a smaller risk, but among these, DiaBeta and Micronase carry the greatest risk due to their slightly longer duration (24 hours versus only 12 to 16 hours for the others). Frequently monitor your blood glucose levels when exercising if you take any of the sulfonylureas that stay in your system for twenty-four hours or longer. As your exercise becomes more regular, check with your doctor or health care provider about lowering your doses of these medications, particularly if you begin to experience hypoglycemia more frequently.

Other medications may affect exercise even less or not at all. Insulin sensitizers like Avandia and Actos influence your at-rest insulin action, so the risk of these medications causing hypoglycemia when you exercise is almost nonexistent. Similarly, Glucophage (metformin) is unlikely to cause exercise lows. Prandin or Starlix only potentially increase your risk of low blood glucose if taken immediately before prolonged exercise, since they increase insulin levels in the blood only temporarily when taken with meals. Finally, medications that slow down the absorption of carbohydrates (Precose and Glyset) don't directly affect exercise but can slightly delay your treatment of a low blood glucose level since you would have to take in carbohydrates to treat it, and thus their absorption would be slowed.

As for injected Symlin and Byetta, few studies have looked at their effects during exercise to date, but exercisers have anecdotally reported that low blood sugar experienced during or following exercise with use of either of these medications is harder to treat (meaning that blood glucose levels do not rise as rapidly in response to glucose or food). Also, some individuals with type 2 diabetes have found that long bouts of exercise are much more difficult with Byetta in their system, which apparently makes them feel more sluggish and less able to do their usual exercise routines.

The myths and the truths about insulin use

The myths and beliefs related to insulin use held by Latinos with diabetes lead many to resist insulin, even when their blood sugar is not well controlled with oral medications. It is critical that you learn the truth about insulin use and tackle your fears about insulin if your doctor recommends it for your diabetes treatment. Insulin may be the best medication for controlling your diabetes, particularly if you have been taking a number of oral pills and they are not doing the job.

Diabetes can result in a progressive loss of insulin-producing beta cells over time, especially if your blood sugar is not well controlled. As a result, your body will be less able to make and release enough insulin to cover your need for it. If you can't make enough of it, you will need to take insulin to compensate.

All people with type 1 diabetes (even slower-onset adults with type 1) and at least 40 percent of people with type 2 must give themselves insulin (be it injected, pumped, or possibly swallowed in the future) to control their blood glucose levels. Being put on insulin if you have type 2 diabetes is not a sign that you have somehow failed or that your diabetes is worse than someone else's. Instead, taking insulin may give your beta cells enough of a rest that they can recover their function.

If your blood sugar is high when your diabetes is discovered (greater than 250 mg/dl, or 13.9 mmol/L), your physician may recommend that you start on insulin immediately. This will allow you to rapidly achieve good control and may have a positive residual effect. Some studies show that when people with type 2 diabetes are started on insulin early, they are unlikely to need supplemental insulin a year later (although they may need it again years down the road). Your insulin dose can then be decreased or withdrawn if your lifestyle changes (e.g., improvements in food, diet, stress management, supplements, and more) control your blood sugar levels in a normal or near normal range. That period of better control when you start using insulin also has a lasting effect when it comes to preventing diabetic complications later on.

If you have type 2 diabetes, your doctor is likely to put you on basal insulin, which covers your non–food related insulin needs and provides stable amounts of insulin during the day. The widely used ones today are Lantus and Levemir, which may be taken once or twice a day. These insulins do not attempt to cover the carbohydrates that you eat during the day, but they help you start the day with better glucose readings and maintain them.

The usual time to onset, peak, and total duration of various insulins are compared in Table 7.4. Three rapid-acting insulin analogs (all synthesized and slightly altered forms of human insulin) are now on the market: Humalog, NovoLog (or Novo-Rapid), and Apidra. Their differences in onset and peak times are minimal, but all are more rapid than the older Regular (e.g., Humulin R) insulin. All of these insulins can be given to cover the food you eat at meals or to correct high blood sugar. Intermediate-action insulins like Humulin N can be used to cover both basal needs and some meals (like lunch), but have become less popular than basal-bolus regimens that better mimic the normal release of insulin from the pancreas. People with type 2 diabetes may also be put on combined insulins containing more of partic-

Table 7.4: The Action of Insulin and Insulin Analogs

Insulin	Onset	Peak	Duration
Humalog/NovoLog/ Apidra	10-30 minutes	0.5-1.5 hours	3-5 hours
Regular (R)	30-60 minutes	2-5 hours	5-8 hours
NPH (N)	1-2 hours	2-12 hours	14-24 hours
Lantus	1.5 hours	None	20-24 hours
Levemir	1-3 hours	8-10 hours	Up to 24 hours

ular basal or intermediate insulins (70 or 75 percent) with some of a rapid-acting one (the other 30 or 25 percent) to cover meal-induced rises in your blood sugar. For many, using combination insulins is an effective therapy. Premixed amounts make it easier for you to take the proper combination of insulin to best cover all of your body's needs. For all injected insulins, smaller doses are generally absorbed from your skin and available in your bloodstream more rapidly than large doses, but smaller amounts also have a shorter duration.

Often when older individuals develop a slower-onset form of type 1 (such as latent autoimmune diabetes of the adult, or LADA), their insulin needs are low for several years, and they may be misdiagnosed as having type 2. Most individuals with type 1, however, require insulin from the start, as oral medications will not effectively treat their condition. The worst thing to do with a child who has rapid-onset type 1 is to put him or her on oral medications rather than insulin. Only insulin will help preserve the remaining insulin-making beta cells in this type of diabetes. The medications used to control the condition may stop working after a while in people who have type 2 diabetes. If you live long enough with diabetes, you will likely need to take supplemental insulin at some point to control your blood sugar, regardless of what type you have.

Should you use syringes, pens, or pumps to take insulin?

To administer insulin, you can use the traditional syringes or the newer insulin pens that hold prefilled insulin cartridges. Using insulin pens reduces the likelihood of giving yourself a dose of the wrong insulin when you use more than one type (and many of the vials look similar) because each insulin has its own unique injection pen. It is also easier to give an exact dose once you dial the dose on a pen, whereas you have to fill a syringe by hand to the correct amount (which can be difficult if you have any visual limitations). If you go on insulin, ask your doctor if he thinks an insulin pen would be easier for you to use than syringes.

Alternatively, you may choose to give insulin to yourself using a specialized insulin pump, which nowadays is about the size of a pager or small cell phone. Pumps utilize a subcutaneous catheter through which small, basal doses of short- or rapid-acting insulin are continually delivered to mimic normal insulin release by the pancreas. You must program the pump to give yourself bolus doses to cover your food intake (mainly carbohydrate) at meals and snacks.

The idea behind insulin pump therapy is to provide insulin just as your body would—in small doses all day long, with bigger doses following food ingestion. This same physiological pattern can be closely mimicked using the newer basal/bolus regimens (e.g., Lantus insulin for basal, Humalog or Novolog for boluses), but insulin pumps make insulin delivery easier and are flexible enough to allow you to change basal rates of insulin delivery at any time. Pump use requires vigilance over your diet and more frequent blood glucose monitoring to catch problems early, but only one needle stick (when the infusion set is inserted) every three to five days for most people. The insulin is directly infused into the skin through the same catheter, which stays under your skin.

Insulin and exercise interactions

If you take insulin, your exercise can cause dramatic effects on your blood sugar. Insulin and muscular contractions evoke separate mechanisms that cause you to take up glucose into muscles, and they additively increase muscle glucose uptake; thus, the type of insulin that you use and the timing of its use can have a large effect on glycemic responses. When no more than basal levels of insulin are circulating in your body during exercise, your body's response will be more normal, as if you didn't have diabetes. If you exercise when your insulin levels are peaking, however, you'll have an increased risk of hypoglycemia. For example, if you inject intermediate-acting N at breakfast, it will peak around noon and exert its effects throughout the afternoon; if you exercise then, your blood glucose level may drop more rapidly than at other times. If you use Lantus or Levemir without any rapid-acting insulin, or your last injection of rapid-acting insulin has peaked and waned before you start exercising, your risk of a low blood glucose level will be much lower. Insulin pump users can normalize exercise responses by either disconnecting their pumps or reducing programmed basal rates during physical activity. Some users also decrease their basal rates before and/or after the activity, depending on how long it lasts and on their individual blood glucose responses.

Other medications with potential effects on exercise

Certain medications (statins) taken to treat high cholesterol levels or abnormal levels of blood fats common in diabetes may result in unexplained muscle pain and weakness with physical activity, possibly by compromising your muscles' ability to generate energy. Luckily, case reports of muscle cramps during or after exercise, nocturnal cramping, and general fatigue suggest that these symptoms resolve when you discontinue taking them. If you are taking a statin and experience any of these symptoms, talk with your doctor about possibly switching to another type of cholesterol-lowering drug.

Medications that reduce the amount of water in your body (diuretics like Lasix, Microzide, Enduron, and Lozol) and improve your blood pressure can lead to dehydration and dizziness from low blood pressure during exercise; they are not likely to affect your blood glucose levels, although they may interfere with insulin secretion. Vasodilators such as nitroglycerin allow more blood to flow to your heart during exercise, but they can also induce hypotension, which may cause you to faint during or following an activity.

You'll also experience a dramatic effect with beta-blockers (e.g., Lopressor, Inderal, Levatol, Corgard, Tenormin, Zebeta) taken to treat heart disease and hypertension, as they lower both resting and exercise heart rate. If you're taking a blocker, your heart rate will not reach an age-expected value at any intensity of exercise, and your ability to reach greater intensity will likely be compromised.

Medications that don't affect exercise

If you take either ACE inhibitors (e.g., Capoten, Accupril, Vasotec, Lotensin, Zestril) or angiotensin II receptor blockers (ARBs, such as Cozaar, Benicar, and Avapro) to reduce your blood pressure and protect your kidneys from possible damage, you should expect no negative effects during exercise. In fact, using certain ACE inhibitors may actually lower your risk of cardiovascular events (like heart attack) if you have heart disease.

Other medications taken to treat heart disease and hypertension (calcium-channel blockers like Procardia, Sular, Cardene, Cardizem, and Norvasc), depression (e.g., Wellbutrin and Prozac), or chronic pain (Celebrex) will have no effect on your ability to exercise. However, keep in mind that aspirin and other blood thinners (such as Coumadin) have the potential to make you bruise more easily or extensively in response to athletic injuries.

CHAPTER 7: *En pocas palabras*

You will benefit greatly from using blood glucose monitoring to determinc your blood sugar response to food, exercise, and more. Try varying the time when you test to manage your blood sugar most effectively. Myriad medications are now available to treat diabetes, including many oral medications for type 2 diabetes and insulins for both type 1 and type 2. Understand the myths about insulin use and embrace using insulin if your doctor recommends it for better diabetes control. Finally, certain medications may affect your response to exercise. Learning how to compensate for a specific medication's effects will allow you to exercise safely, regardless of which medications you take.

CHAPTER 8

Controlling Stress, Depression, and Your Emotions

Nowadays, no one questions the importance of a positive mental outlook in making permanent health changes and forming optimal habits for lifelong wellness. Many in the Latino community control stress and depression and keep a positive outlook by relying on interactions with family and community support systems. Effectively managing your emotional state is important because stress and depression can have a negative effect on blood sugar control, and possibly on the development of diabetes in the first place. In this chapter we talk about why this is the case and examine the impact of physical activity and food on your mood and mental outlook. We'll also address dieting and why it tends to be unhealthy.

Why keeping a positive outlook and managing stress matter

Many people who live successfully with diabetes insist that a positive attitude is one of the key secrets to living well with diabetes, avoiding

Tips for Relaxing and Reducing Your Stress

- Spend several minutes doing deep breathing—slowly inhaling and exhaling—and visualize emotional stress leaving your body.
- Sit quietly and imagine that you are in a calm, restful place, such as at the beach, in the woods, or with a group of close friends—whatever works for you.
- Meditate by sitting quietly (preferably with your eyes closed), breathing slowly and deeply, and focusing all of your thoughts on a single image in your mind, object in the room, or sound for ten to twenty minutes.
- Use progressive muscle relaxation, tensing an area of your body first and then fully relaxing it, starting at your toes and working up your whole body.
- Listen to soothing music, relaxation tapes, or CDs that you enjoy.
- Practice self-hypnosis, which is like meditation but uses positive affirmation. For example, you may repeat a mantra, such as "I have a healthy body" or "I am in control of my diabetes."
- Do yoga exercise and yoga deep breathing regularly.
- Go out for a brisk walk or just get up and move around for a few minutes.
- Socialize with family and friends to get your mind off your perceived problems.

depression, and feeling happy overall. Current research confirms that attitude matters. For example, a recent forty-year study following students who attended the University of North Carolina in the mid-1960s found that pessimists had a 42 percent higher death rate from all causes compared with optimists, who were less likely to suffer from depression. Being depressed may actually contribute to the onset of diabetes and other chronic disorders (more on this later).

Is it possible to manage emotional stress? Research indicates that it is. For instance, a five-session group stress management program in a real-world setting was found to reduce stress and improve diabetes control for people with type 2 diabetes. Thus it's both important and possible for you to learn how to control the effect that stress has on your mental and physical condition. There are a number of things you can do to reduce stress, including simple things like taking slow, deep breaths, or laughing. In people with diabetes, research shows, laughing can lower blood pressure and possibly after-meal spikes in blood glucose. Laughter is definitely good medicine: Being able to laugh in stressful situations may also lower your risk of developing heart disease.

Although about 50 percent of your capacity to feel happy and minimize worry may be attributable to your genes (i.e., your inherited personality), the other half is under your control. Being grateful for what you have and connecting with others socially are apparently the most important factors in avoiding depression and reaching a higher level of happiness, which is especially important in dealing with diabetes. Feeling happy reduces your stress level, leading to better self-care, fewer indulgent behaviors, and greater adherence to daily exercise and food plans. Engaging in negative thought patterns and dwelling on the bad things in your life are surefire ways to stay unhappy.

You are the only one with the capacity to change your thoughts for the better. If you are feeling a negative emotion, acknowledge it and then replace it with a positive one. You even have the power to change how you view having diabetes, from a downer to an upper. You could choose to feel depressed over the fact that it's currently an incurable condition, but you will likely feel better about your diabetes and your life in general if you use all the tools at your disposal to control your blood glucose levels and conquer it on your own. At least you'll be taking positive steps to control the things that you can influence and letting go of the things that you can't. Doing so will make you a happier person.

You can help yourself become more optimistic by practicing strategies like anger management and meditation to boost positive emotions. Researchers who studied Tibetan Buddhist monks, many of whom have spent over 10,000 hours in meditation, found evidence that a positive state of mind is a skill that can be learned through training, much as the monks have done with hours of focused thought. It appears that the conscious act of thinking about your thoughts in a particular way can rearrange your brain, chemically speaking. If nothing else, putting on a sunny face regardless of how you really feel can actually alter your mood for the better by affecting your thought patterns.

Does stress really cause gray hairs and diabetes?

A recent study found accelerated aging in the DNA of mothers caring for children who had life-threatening diseases like cancer. It is possible that excessive or prolonged emotional stress can give you more gray hairs or drive you to an early grave. Stress has a major influence on your circulatory system, and it plays a significant role in susceptibility to, progress in, and outcome of cardiovascular disease.

Not all stress is bad, but emotional stress due to diabetes or other chronic illnesses is likely more detrimental than helpful. Any stress (e.g., making it through the holiday season) can suppress your body's immune function and increase your likelihood of getting sick—even with the common cold—by increasing your cortisol levels. Compound that level of stress day after day by living with diabetes and throw depression into the mix, and it's easy to understand why people with diabetes need to learn how to control their stress levels before they further negatively affect their physical health. What's more, mental or physical stress can cause a rise in both adrenaline and cortisol levels, both of which decrease insulin action and make diabetes management more difficult. Excess levels of cortisol are also at least partially responsible for low-level systemic inflammation, which may be the link between depression and the development of type 2 diabetes.

Emotional concerns arising from diabetes or your weight

Regardless of how you responded to your diagnosis of type 2 diabetes (and possibly other concurrent health conditions), you likely have special emotional concerns that often arise in those dealing with an "incurable" chronic health condition. No one feels good about being put down for being overweight or having diabetes. It's a reality for many people, though. Diabetes is a less obvious condition than being overweight because it can be hidden (as many in the Latino community have traditionally done). Being denigrated, maligned, or discriminated against because of your body weight can easily play into and worsen feelings of low self-esteem that you may have or even lead to feelings of helplessness and depression. A Finnish study found a positive relationship between insulin resistance and serious depressive symptoms (an association that was already present in people with prediabetes), so it's very likely that being depressed can accelerate the onset of diabetes.

Latinos may not always recognize or treat depression

In the United States, about one adult in ten has major depressive disorder (the most serious form), but it's more than twice as common among people with diabetes. Almost half of all people with diabetes have either major or milder forms of depression, particularly if they have other health problems like heart disease, chronic arthritis, and stroke. Mood disorders, including depression, cross all national, cultural, ethnic, and gender boundaries. Particularly in the Latino community, where traditional gender roles may further contribute to an unwillingness to talk about feelings of depression, unrecognized and untreated depression is a serious concern. According to the National Latino and Asian American Study, 54 percent of Latino men with at least one episode of major depression in their lifetime do not recognize having a mental health problem. In addition, Latinos are reluctant to get treatment for depression, and Latino men are afraid that seeking treatment will endanger their job. Men with depression, regardless of ethnic background, may be more likely to turn to alcohol or drugs, or to become frustrated, angry, or irritable instead of acknowledging their feelings and asking for help as women tend to do. Some men may throw themselves into their work or hobbies to hide their depression from themselves, family, and friends, while others may engage in reckless behavior that leads to poor self-care.

Physical health and mental health are interrelated, and your physical well-being often can't be improved if your psychological problems are not addressed. When you are depressed, you may feel sad and hopeless and you may lose interest in things you normally enjoy. You may also eat or sleep much more or less than usual, have low energy levels, have trouble concentrating, and feel bad about yourself. Depression also increases the likelihood that you will die in the next ten years if you have diabetes. Out of more than five hundred people with diabetes, according to a recent study, the depressed ones had a 54 percent greater mortality rate. Latinos who remain depressed are also more likely to have declining cognitive function over time. Effective treatments for depression are available, however, and the success rate is high among people who seek help and remain in treatment.

MANNY HERNANDEZ
Sharing his diabetes on TuDiabetes.com and EsTuDiabetes.com

Manuel "Manny" Hernandez has been living with diabetes since 2002, and he has made his mark on the way that people with diabetes communicate with each other around the world—looking for friendship, emotional support, networking, and knowledge about diabetes. He was diagnosed at the age of thirty. Initially, because of his age and excess body weight (240 pounds), he was told that he had type 2 diabetes. "Over time, the typical oral treatments that work for type 2 were not working for me anymore, so I was referred to an endocrinologist," he states. "I tested positive for antibodies in my blood associated with type 1 diabetes, and my C-peptide levels were on the floor," indicating that he was not producing his own insulin. "So I was diagnosed as type 1 in early 2003." His experience with diabetes onset is quite common in adults who develop type 1.

For Manny, making healthier lifestyle choices was the easy part. "I immediately adjusted my lifestyle and started eating healthier meals and exercising," he recalls. He tries to restrict his carbohydrate intake at each meal to less than 60 grams, following a diet with no more than 40 percent of calories from carbohydrates, and he's physically active. "I walk and bike," he says. "I don't do it every day because my schedule is super hectic, but try to make sure I incorporate it into my routine every week. Also, I make a point of getting extra activity by parking far from places I go and taking the stairs whenever I can."

Going off oral medications and starting on insulin was a challenge for him, though. He was used to taking pills for being sick or vitamins as a supplement, but having to take shots was something else. "While I wasn't happy to find out I had type 2, it was less of a shock than dealing with insulin shots for type 1 later on," he admits. "When I had to start with insulin, it took much more adjusting. Syringes are not an everyday thing, so it was rough initially. I think young people who grow up with type 1, having to take shots, normally do better than adults having to start injecting. However, as with everything, you end up getting used to it." Before he finally started using an insulin pump, he was taking eight shots a day. Switching to one needle prick every three days to insert the pump's infusion set was an easy decision for him.

Manny believes that having diabetes is not a death sentence and does not have to result in diabetes-related health complications. "However," he says, "you have to help yourself to make sure this is the case." He thinks that the main barriers that diabetic Latinos face when it comes to diabetes care are misinformation, language and cultural barriers (particularly for Latinos in the United States), and genetics. His family does a lot to help him deal with his diabetes. "My wife is my biggest ally in the daily management of my diabetes. She is not the 'diabetes police'; she knows how to balance her input very well in ways that are not annoying but helpful. She does most of the cooking," Manny says, "but my son and I are helpers in the kitchen. I love the plates she prepares, and she loves healthy eating too, so it's not hard to do for either one of us."

Interacting with others in the Latino diabetes community has helped Manny tremendously. As he recalls, "Back in 2006, I started attending an insulin pumpers club in Orlando, Florida, where we used to live. That group taught me lots of things and exposed me for the first time to a group of other people with diabetes in a way that was very influential. Having so many people together that 'got me' allowed me to feel understood and welcomed in so many ways. I also learned a ton from them." Following that experience, he got the idea of founding a social network for Latinos and others with diabetes. In March 2007 he and others launched TuDiabetes.com, a "community for people touched by diabetes" that is open to people with diabetes, their family members and friends, and others. Later that year, they launched EsTuDiabetes.com, a sister community only in Spanish since they realized that people who speak little English need to connect with others in their own language. In 2008 he and others additionally launched the Diabetes Hands Foundation, a nonprofit organization that aims to connect people who have diabetes and raise awareness about it.

To live well with diabetes, Manny says that first you need to accept your disease. Then you need to educate yourself about diabetes and ask questions. He also finds it helpful to love himself—despite having diabetes—and to connect with others with diabetes to reinforce this. "Diabetes can be a very tough condition and even tougher if you live with it all by yourself," he says. "Not only does meeting others help with coping with hard times, but also it can give you lots of tools and tips you can incorporate into your daily managements so that you can 'fill in the gaps' between doctor visits."

Emotional fitness through physical activity

Exercise is vitally important in alleviating feelings of stress, anxiety, and depression. Anyone can use regular exercise to relieve mild to moderate symptoms of depression and anxiety and improve mood and self-concept. Being physically active, particularly if you are prone to depression, allows you to experience better mental and physical health and less depression. It can also positively affect your self-perceptions, benefiting your self-confidence, self-concept, and self-esteem. Especially for women and girls, bodily dissatisfaction is associated with lower self-esteem. If you perceive yourself as fat and out of shape, you'll be particularly vulnerable to a negative self-image. Exercise can improve your body shape and size, raise your self-esteem, and improve your bodily satisfaction. Finally, in addition to improving your short-term mental state and mood, exercise promotes an overall sense of well being.

As for physical health, your cortisol levels rise when your blood glucose levels are not well controlled. The result is that you become even more insulin resistant, your pancreatic beta cells have to work even harder, and your glucose control can worsen over time. Luckily, this vicious cycle is best reversed by regular physical activity. Once you begin to exercise, your energy levels are likely to rise and your physical health will improve. Feeling better physically will improve your mental outlook and likely improve your ability to manage your diabetes.

One of the emotional benefits of exercise is the release of hormones in your brain called endorphins, mood-enhancing hormones that bind to natural receptors and cause feelings of euphoria after you have been exercising for a while (producing a "second wind"). There is evidence that endorphins may actually improve your body's insulin action, thereby reversing or decreasing insulin resistance as well. In fact, endorphin release may be a major mechanism in the enhanced insulin sensitivity attributable to moderate exercise. Aim to release endorphins and other mood-enhancing brain hormones on a daily basis through physical activity to control your blood sugar and improve your outlook at the same time.

Maybe you need to get a pet for better health

Researchers investigating the fitness of dog walkers versus people who work out at a gym (the study was funded by a dog food company) found that walking a dog daily lowered owners' blood pressure, slowed their heart rates, reduced stress, and resulted in quicker recovery from strenuous activity. Of the 1,500 people studied, the average dog walker covered a distance of 676 miles a year, which was over 200 miles more than gym goers. More importantly, most dog owners continued with their daily walking routine, whereas more than half of gym goers dropped out of their programs after two or three months. Thus owning a dog that has to be walked, regardless of the weather, may keep you more active and healthy.

Another positive benefit for dog owners is that having to walk their pet regularly increases social contact, which for many people enhances their feelings of happiness and social connectedness—especially Latinos who value a sense of community more than other ethnic groups do. Pets can be a conversation starter that leads to greater social interactions. Studies have also demonstrated that interactions with pets can lower anxiety and reduce stress, which can benefit your blood sugar control. If you are a cat lover, sitting with a purring cat on your lap may be enough to change your outlook from negative to positive. Even watching tropical fish swim in a tank can bring about a sense of relaxation. If nothing else, having a pet to care for helps take your focus off yourself and your own health for at least a few minutes a day. Whatever type of pet works best to alleviate your stress and improve your health should be the one you get.

Stay mentally active

You can prevent declines in memory and mental functioning. All you need to do is eat better, exercise more, control your diabetes, smoke less, and challenge your mind. Whether that means you take a dance class, learn another language, practice memory exercises, or do daily crossword puzzles, you'll be much less likely to suffer from declining mental capacity in your later years. Even if your mental processes already seem to be declining, you can reverse the trend. For example, elderly people who go through training to improve the sharpness of their thinking and challenge their memory score much better on thinking tests for years afterward, and even young people who drill their memories have minds that work more efficiently.

You will benefit most from engaging in a rich diversity of stimulating activities. New experiences may be more important than repeating the same task over and over; try combining mental stimulation with social interaction for the greatest benefit. Most of all, enjoy the activities you take part in, because stress and other negative emotions appear to be harmful to your mental ability (not to mention your blood glucose control). Even relaxation techniques

---

Mental Exercises to Maintain a Better Mental Function

- Practice memorizing anything and recall it later.
- Observe an object and then later draw it from memory.
- Draw a map of places you have visited after you return home.
- Play card or board games that require mental reasoning, such as pinochle, bridge, chess, checkers, Othello, or Lotería (a Mexican game similar to Bingo, but using images on a deck of cards).
- Do daily crossword puzzles, anagrams, Sudoku, and other word or reasoning games.
- Play video games, particularly the fast-moving ones that require quick reactions.
- Listen to or read the news and then write out a summary.
- Try to do something new or unusual every day that requires you to think.
- Practice doing math problems in your head instead of with a calculator.
- Learn a new language, either on your own or by taking a class.
- Read a lot of different types of things, including fiction and nonfiction.

---

may benefit your mental functioning for that reason. For some older Latinos, attending church moderates symptoms of depression, which in turn helps maintain their cognitive abilities.

The effect of food on your mood

Latino cultures are not the only ones that focus on food in social interactions. It's true that certain foods affect your mood by causing the release of various brain hormones that can actually soothe anxiety and depression, but using them to change your mood only works up to a point. If you indulge in chocolate or fatty foods to raise your mood, you may end up feeling guilty about the resulting rise in your blood sugar or body weight. Likewise, eating sugar and consuming caffeine to alter your mood is at best a temporary mood enhancer, which more often than not is followed by a crash. Moreover, the latest research indicates that sugar may be addictive—possibly even more so than heroin and cocaine—because it causes the release of brain hormones like dopamine that your brain craves when deprived of carbohydrate intake. Replace this addiction with exercise instead and avoid such crashes and lapses in self-control.

As far as emotional benefits are concerned, some foods have a longer-term positive effect, including foods high in omega-3 fatty acids (e.g., fish and many nuts), which are also good for the health of your cardiovascular system. Healthy carbohydrates found in whole fruits that have fiber, vitamins, minerals, and phytonutrients also can have a soothing effect. But remember to eat everything in moderation. Although you may crave them, do your best to avoid bingeing on refined carbohydrates (processed foods) that cause rapid spikes in your blood sugar. To help your metabolism run more smoothly, take in enough B vitamins, particularly folate, niacin, B6, and B12, which are found in abundance in high-fiber carbohydrate foods like legumes.

Your choice of foods may also alter your capacity to reason, remember, and function mentally. If you are overweight or used to be, your risk of developing dementia at some point in your life is higher, and having prediabetes or diabetes also increases your chances of both Alzheimer's disease and dementia. The link may be damage from free radicals, which is where foods rich in antioxidants come in. Such foods also help prevent plaque formation in the arteries that feed your heart and your brain and thereby help prevent heart attack and stroke.

Your relationship with food and disordered eating

Most dysfunctional relationships with food, or eating disorders, originate with dieting. About half a million people in the United

States are battling eating disorders, such as bingeing and purging, compulsive overeating, or self-starvation, at any given time. Adults suffering from such disorders range from the underweight to the morbidly obese, but many are normal weight individuals too. Health care professionals are finally realizing that dieting is not a viable long-term solution to weight control for most people and that forced diets encourage the development of dysfunctional eating habits and obsessions over food and body weight. Your goal should be simply to achieve and maintain good health and prevent yourself from gaining more weight.

If you are overweight and have diabetes, you are likely to have some form of disordered eating, given that you're probably struggling to gain or maintain control over both your body weight and your blood glucose levels. You may have simply stopped eating as much as usual or become much choosier about foods to self-impose a diet. If you start eating again after consuming a full meal, you may be doing so out of sadness, boredom, or depression. You may eat and drink too much at social gatherings just because you don't want to stand out or be different. In addition, elevated blood glucose levels create a drive to eat that has nothing to do with true hunger.

Although binge-eating disorders are more prevalent in diabetic individuals, breaking your abstinence from forbidden treats with overindulgence is similar to falling off the wagon with drug or alcohol abuse. Don't beat yourself up so badly that you lose your motivation to resume your more healthful regimens. As long as you get back on the better nutrition wagon, your good intentions will not have been for naught. Seek out assistance to deal with your altered emotional relationship with food—carbohydrates in particular—and better diabetes control will naturally follow.

Moderation is the key

To eradicate type 2 diabetes, we Latinos (and everyone else) must learn, both individually and as a community, to stop "supersizing" our desires. However, complete abstinence from favorite treats is not the best way to approach lifelong eating changes. To maintain a life-long, healthy meal plan, as we advocate, you don't need to completely abstain from any food. You can allow yourself to have small amounts of the foods that you really enjoy, and take your time eating them to maximize your enjoyment. In fact, you can eat anything your heart desires—but you must learn to consume unhealthier foods in moderation. Your interpretation of moderation needs to be revisited occasionally to keep it honest. A good rule of thumb is that if the item you are eating is a high-GI, high-GL food, you should limit your intake to no more than one small serving per day.

If you find yourself faced with a buffet-style meal or food-oriented social gathering, you can still maintain control. Start with a full plate of salad (but go easy on the dressing) or green vegetables. Wait at least ten to fifteen minutes, and then return for a second, smaller plateful of main course "samples." Use smaller plates if they're available, never go back for a third helping, eat slowly, drink plenty of water or calorie-free beverages, and stop eating before you feel full.

Practice makes perfect when it comes to eating the right amount

You will likely have to practice moderating your eating to learn how to do it. If you're having a high-GI dessert like flan or bread pudding, serve yourself half of your normal amount on a smaller plate (to make it look larger) and take twice as long as usual to eat it. Really, it's the first couple of bites that taste the best, and you will feel just as satisfied after eating the smaller quantity (not to mention less guilty) if you really enjoy it. Slower eating allows all of your senses to experience and enjoy the flavor, while allowing your stomach to register its fullness in conscious regions of your brain.

Not only should you eat desserts more slowly, but you should also slow down on finishing the rest of your meal. Stop eating when you are about 80 percent full (or at least leave a few bites on your plate), and you'll feel 100 percent satisfied after a short while instead of overly stuffed. Drinking water or other beverages before a meal or starting with broth-based soup also helps make you feel full before you eat as much. If you eat quickly, wait at least ten minutes (preferably fifteen to twenty) after finishing your first (moderate) helping before going back for seconds (during which time your stomach may register its fullness). You might even plan to eat a light snack two to three hours after your meal instead of overeating.

Involve your familia *and others in your diabetes care*

Maintaining a special meal plan, exercising regularly, keeping stress levels low, and feeling good about diabetes is hard to accomplish on your own. Most long-timers with diabetes agree that a supportive husband, wife, significant other, family, and friends are crucial to managing diabetes and living well. Studies confirm that connecting with others around you is one of the most important factors in avoiding depression as well as reaching a higher level of happiness, which can keep you from stressing and overindulging in comfort foods that may raise your blood sugar.

Although family and friends usually mean well, sometimes their support can be smothering. When you involve your family

EMMA FERNANDEZ SILVA
AND SOCORRO CIENFUEGOS
Making diabetes a family affair

Immigrants to the United States from Mexico, Emma Fernandez Silva and Socorro Cienfuegos have shown that having diabetes can be a family affair. Emma recently passed away at the age of ninety-one after living with type 2 diabetes for more than forty-two years, with lots of assistance from her daughter and other family members in her later years. Socorro recalls that physical activity was always a big part of her mother's life. "My mother walked every day since she lacked transportation where she lived in Mexico until 1998. She also liked to bowl and ice skate," and continued to do both through most of her life. Mother and daughter both believed that lack of daily activity is a big part of the diabetes problem in Latino communities in their native country and other Hispanic ones.

Even though *hija* Socorro had watched her mother live with diabetes for many years before she herself was diagnosed with it at the age of fifty-four, she had a hard time accepting the diagnosis. "I was in denial at first," Socorro recalls. "I started consuming more of everything that my doctor had forbidden and gained more weight. My doctor forbade me from eating almost all fruits, leaving me only with vegetables. I was prohibited from eating a normal diet, which gave me the image of having a catastrophic disease rather than a treatable one."

Once she began to inform herself about diabetes, though, she was able to get it under control with a modified diet and medication. Nowadays, she eats a healthy diet with plenty of vegetables (including squash, cauliflower, cabbage, carrots, corn, tomatoes, onions, and garlic), balanced out with some fruit, brown rice, beans without oil, lentils and broad beans, bread, and chicken. Just as important as a healthy diet is the walk that she takes every day and the exercise she does at her gym in Chulavista, California, for an hour twice a week.

Madre Emma had a strong family history of diabetes. Her father died from gangrene in his leg related to the disease, and all of her brothers have it along with senile dementia. Not only does *hija* Socorro have type

2 diabetes, but so does her brother, who has lost sight related to poor control of the disease. Socorro has learned that having good control of blood sugar is the key to preventing diabetes-related problems, having seen the evidence in her own life and health, as well as in her family's. Her daughter developed gestational diabetes but was able to control her blood sugar and gave birth to a perfectly healthy, seven-pound baby girl in the spring of 2008.

Asked what would help Latinos take on the diabetes *problema* more effectively, she says, "It would be helpful to have more educators who can explain about the foods in a Hispanic diet and in an American one that are good for people with diabetes—in Spanish." She has found the lack of information in Spanish to be hard, along with the great quantity of American foods with lots of sugar, and limited time to exercise when caring for her own family (Emma before her death, and Socorro's own children). To live well with diabetes, she believes that people need to be more physically active, eat a healthier diet (with lots of vegetables and fruits), drink more water, learn more about alternative medicine options and preventive strategies, manage stress better, and realize that Latinos need to make some changes in their way of living to prevent diabetes in their children and teenagers.

members and close friends in your diabetes care, make sure they also know when to back off and stop hovering. If someone says to you, "You can't eat that—you have diabetes!" use it as an opportunity to share what you have learned about managing diabetes rather than feeling offended or smothered by the criticism.

Finally, having someone important in your life who also has diabetes—a friend, hero, or mentor—can make all the difference in how well you take care of yourself. Try to spend time with others who have diabetes on a regular basis and share your frustrations and your successes. Alternately, sometimes it's beneficial to be someone else's hero, to give him or her someone to look up to or admire. Once you feel confident in managing your diabetes, share your wealth of knowledge with others who are just learning the ropes. You may learn a thing or two more about yourself along the way.

CHAPTER 8: *En pocas palabras*

Stress and depression can have a negative effect on blood sugar control, possibly contributing to the development of diabetes in the first place, so maintaining a positive outlook helps you manage your diabetes more effectively. Latinos may not always recognize depression and seek out treatment, though. Becoming physically active can benefit your emotional state and your mental fitness. Food also affects your mood, but disordered eating can be a problem for individuals who have focused repeatedly on dieting unless they learn to be moderate in their eating. Finally, to ensure your emotional health (and better physical health as a result), invite your family and friends to be a part of your diabetes care team.

CHAPTER 9

Limiting Diabetes-Related Health Problems

How seriously do people with diabetes consider their condition to be? Recently focus group participants were asked to rank the severity of various health problems, including cancer, heart disease, and diabetes. On a scale of one to ten, cancer and heart disease consistently ranked at or near the top of the scale for severity, while diabetes only scored fours and fives. However, diabetes is a serious disease not to be taken lightly. Perhaps it is ranked lower than other diseases because there is medication to treat it. People usually die of diabetes-related complications like heart attacks, where diabetes is not necessarily recognized as the underlying cause of death.

In fact diabetes is anything but minor as far as your health is concerned. This disease has the potential to wreak havoc on your entire body, affecting everything from hearing and vision to sexual function, mental health, sleep, and cardiovascular health. Poorly controlled diabetes is the leading cause of blindness, amputation, and kidney failure in the United States, and it can triple your risk for heart attack and stroke. As one diabetes researcher said, "It is a disease that does have the ability to eat you alive." Unfortunately, diabetes-related health complications are a reality for many people living with the disease. You need to understand what causes them, what symptoms to look out for, and how to prevent them in the first place.

What you need to know about possible diabetic complications

As you have learned in this book, you can live *la vida buena* despite having diabetes. To help you achieve this, we're going to revisit the list of possible diabetes complications, not to depress or scare you but to help you understand that what you choose to do can make a difference in preventing them.

On average, diabetes has the potential to rob you of more than twelve years of life while dramatically reducing your quality of life for more than twenty years—through partial limb amputations, chronic pain, loss of mobility, blindness, chronic dialysis, and heart disease. Experts recently estimated that for the 38.5 percent of average females (or more, if you're Latina) born in 2000 or later predicted to develop diabetes, the disease will shorten their lives by over fourteen years (if diagnosed by the age of 40) and make their lives less worth living during the last twenty-two of those years. As far as we're concerned, feeling good while you are alive and being able to do everything you want to do is far more important than living a long life filled with suffering from diabetic complications, most of which are preventable. Showing you that you can prevent health problems by controlling your diabetes and teaching you how to do it is the main purpose of this book.

We all want to live a long life, as long as we are healthy, vital, and energetic. Having diabetes, however, gives you twice the risk of dying as someone who is diabetes-free. If you're a younger type 2 diabetic individual (between 25 and 44), your risk is almost four times as high. Diabetes is the sixth leading cause of death, but it should actually have a higher ranking. Why? If you die from a heart attack or stroke, your death certificate may not even mention diabetes as a cause or contributing factor, even though we now know that poor blood sugar control accelerates the blockage of arteries around your body. Diabetes is a direct or indirect cause of more than 3.2 million deaths per year around the world, and this statistic is only going to get gloomier in the near future unless we all collectively take the steps necessary to prevent it. *¡Qué problema!*

Individually, heart disease and stroke are the most common cardiovascular diseases (CVD), which often lead to a lower quality of life, an older biological age (meaning that your body has aged more than normally expected for someone of your chronological age), and a shortened life span. More than 70 million Americans currently live with some form of CVD. Although these health conditions are more common among people over sixty-five, the number of sudden deaths from heart disease among people between fifteen and thirty-four has recently increased, with declines in health attributable to poor lifestyle choices. If unhealthy lifestyles are causing such problems, then it stands to reason that they can be prevented or reversed by improving diet and increasing physical activity.

Diabetes can accelerate the development of heart and other vascular diseases. The leading cause of death in all Americans is the same for people with diabetes: heart disease. If you have diabetes, though, your risk of dying from a heart attack is elevated. Many undiagnosed people with type 2 diabetes first learn of their condition shortly after having their first heart attack. At that point, they likely have had diabetes for years without knowing it, but long enough for it to cause significant damage. Ignorance of diabetes is certainly not bliss, but about one-quarter of all people with type 2 diabetes remain undiagnosed even though their elevated blood sugar is doing damage. Cardiovascular problems are very common in type 2 diabetes, but their incidence can be reduced significantly with blood sugar control. For those with type 1 diabetes, intensive diabetes management has also been shown to reduce their risk of cardiovascular disease.

Plaque buildup in the coronary arteries begins in childhood, and when you have other commonly occurring health problems, like high blood pressure and elevated cholesterol levels to go along with diabetes, heart disease can progress more rapidly. Unfortunately, almost three-fourths of adults with diabetes have high blood pressure (with readings above 140 over 90 mm Hg) that may not be effectively controlled with medication, and most have abnormal levels of blood fats and cholesterol.

Elevated blood sugar levels can damage your eyes, kidneys, and nerves, leading to proliferative retinopathy, nephropathy, and neuropathy. People with diabetes are twenty-five times more likely to go blind. Poorly controlled diabetes can lead to the onset of proliferative diabetic retinopathy, a severe form of diabetic eye disease that can cause hemorrhaging into the eye, vision loss, and retinal detachment. It causes tens of thousands of new cases of blindness annually, only some of which are reversible with surgical removal and replacement of the vitreous fluid inside the eye. In addition, diabetes causes six other types of eye disease that can negatively impact your vision, including glaucoma, cataracts, macular degeneration, and neuropathy of the optic nerves.

Your kidneys can be similarly affected by diabetes, which is the leading cause of new cases of kidney disease requiring dialysis and ultimately kidney transplants. In many cases, progression of kidney disease can be delayed with medications that protect kidney function, but you want to detect it as early as possible for the best results.

Traditionally, 60 to 70 percent of diabetic individuals also experience mild to severe nerve damage. Symptoms include impaired sensation (numbness) or shooting pains (painful neuropathy) in feet or hands, gastroparesis (slowing of the digestion that can cause symptoms like nausea, vomiting, bloating, abdominal pain, heartburn, and alternating diarrhea and constipation), orthostatic hypertension (severe dizziness when standing up), and even erectile dysfunction in men and decreased sexual function in women. Diabetic ulcers, often related to nerve damage in the feet and lower limbs, cause the majority of over 40,000 annual toe, foot, and leg amputations in the United States. In men who have yet to be diagnosed with diabetes, erectile dysfunction is often a symptom of diabetes and vascular problems.

Diabetes has been linked with many other potential health problems as well, including hearing loss, joint problems, poor pregnancy outcomes, increased risk of miscarriage, and more. By now, you should understand that diabetes is a disease to be reckoned with, and you must control it effectively before it has a chance to take control of you.

Latinos have it worse when it comes to complications

Compared with the rest of the population, Latinos are twice as likely to suffer from severe diabetic complications. Deaths from diabetes among Latino populations are more than double the proportion of diabetes-related deaths in non-Latinos. This disease is the sixth leading cause of death in Latino communities, but the fourth leading cause of death among Latino women and elders. If you are Latino and have diabetes, your risk for having severe retinopathy is greater than for your white counterparts, and it may occur at an earlier age. Other complications occur earlier and are more severe in Latino populations as well.

What explains the worse outcome for Latinos? One recent study suggested that some of the disparity could be due to Latinos' greater difficulty in controlling diabetes: Their A1c values are typically 0.5 percent higher than in other populations. It may also have to do with socioeconomic factors such as limited access to quality health care, because the individuals with the highest average blood sugar were those with the poorest access to health care. These findings suggest that with better care and earlier intervention, the complication rates for Latinos could be lowered significantly.

Living la vida buena *with diabetes and preventing diabetic complications*

How do you go about living *la vida buena* with diabetes? Many studies have shown that modifying your lifestyle, at any age, has a powerful effect on maintaining your health and your physical function. Managing your body weight, not smoking, controlling your blood pressure and blood sugar, and exercising regularly are all linked to an enhanced life span, good health, and better function as you age.

You can learn how to prevent and control diabetic health problems before they occur, largely by developing good health habits early on to prevent complications. Preventing problems and then controlling any that do arise involves finding out about the latest treatment and technologies available. In Chapter 4, we mentioned herbal and other nonprescription treatments for certain complications, but medical treatments may be even more effective, used alone or in combination with certain supplements. For example, controlling the progression of kidney disease involves the use of ACE-inhibitors, blood pressure medications, and better methods to keep your blood sugar in an optimal range. Either ACE-inhibitors (angiotensin-converting enzyme inhibitors) or another class of drugs known as ARBs (angiotensin receptor blockers) can slow early kidney disease by 30 to 70 percent. With such aggressive treatments, many individuals avoid end-stage kidney problems, including dialysis and kidney transplants. Have both your albumin levels (in your urine) and your blood creatinine levels measured annually to detect kidney disease early, when it can usually be controlled. Although high protein diets are not likely to cause kidney problems, limiting protein if you develop kidney damage is prudent.

Certain complications like gastroparesis, which slows your stomach emptying after a meal, make it harder to control blood sugar after eating. Slow carbohydrate absorption can cause low blood sugar after eating and taking insulin, with hyperglycemia developing later on. If you have severe gastroparesis, try to limit your carbohydrate intake to 80 grams or less a day (about 30 per meal) to make your blood sugar easier to control. Likewise, eating small quantities of food at one time will help keep food moving through your stomach and intestines. Some people use Reglan, a prescription medication, to relieve the symptoms.

Other peripheral nerve problems can cause pain or numbness in your feet and legs and occasionally arms and hands, which may be controllable with medications like Cymbalta, Neurontin, and Lyrica. Some individuals experience side effects with their use; for example, both Cymbalta and Neurontin, used to treat painful neuropathy, can cause dizziness, so talk with your doctor if you have any symptoms while taking them. Interestingly, recent studies of diabetic people doing long-term aerobic exercise training found that it may prevent the onset or slow the progression of peripheral nerve damage, so exercising by itself may be a good preventative medicine for many.

To care for your eyes and detect changes early, when problems are more easily treated, have a dilated eye exam performed at least annually, ideally by an ophthalmologist (not an optometrist). When people with diabetes go blind, it's because they didn't visit an eye doctor until too late. Nowadays blindness is preventable. If you develop diabetes in childhood, you should have your eyes checked by the time you reach puberty (around age thirteen). Anyone else who is diagnosed with diabetes should have an eye exam right away. If your sight is reduced from hemorrhages inside your eyes caused by the growth of unstable new vessels (proliferative retinopathy), treatment usually consists of laser burns to the peripheral parts of the back of the eye (retina), along with a vitrectomy to surgically remove the cloudy vitreous fluid in your eyes if it fails to clear out on its own. These treatments restore central vision in many individuals. The sooner you catch and treat these changes in the eye, the more successful the treatment is likely to be.

Cardiovascular health issues can be controlled through early intervention; dietary and exercise interventions; medications to control blood pressure and cholesterol levels; angioplasty; placement of arterial stents (to open up coronary arteries); bypass surgery, and more. Aspirin therapy is also recommended for most adults with diabetes, along with smoking cessation. In the case of vascular problems, early intervention—before you have a heart attack or stroke—can greatly lower your chances of dying early or having debilitating health problems, so get checked out regularly, particularly if you start to experience symptoms of reduced blood flow to any part of your body. Chest pain at rest or during exertion, shortness of breath, and pain in your legs during walking (i.e., peripheral vascular changes) are all potential signs of problems that you should have checked as soon as possible.

A sudden loss of vision, a sudden inability to walk or stand, or a sudden slurring of your words can be symptoms of a stroke, and you should be seen immediately by a physician. If you experience a stroke and can get to a hospital within three hours from the onset of symptoms to receive a clot-busting drug called tPA, your outcome is much more likely to be favorable. Antiplatelet agents, such as aspirin and Plavix, and anticoagulants like Coumadin interfere with the blood's ability to clot and can play an important role in preventing stroke. However, if you have stomach ulcers or already take other anti-inflammatory drugs like Advil, you should take no more than a baby aspirin (81 mg) a day; for others, 325 mg of a coated aspirin like Ecotrin may be a more effective stroke preventative.

People with diabetes are also more likely to develop periodontal (gum) disease, and good oral hygiene can help prevent problems before they start. While poor oral hygiene is a factor in gum disease for everyone, having diabetes accelerates the process, and poorly controlled blood sugar is the main cause of gum disease among adults. Circulatory problems linked to diabetes can make your gums more susceptible to infections, which can in turn lead to inflammation of the gums and loss of gum tissue. High glucose levels in saliva also promote the growth of bacteria on teeth and gums and plaque formation. Periodontal problems that develop under these conditions have been linked to a higher incidence of heart disease and strokes.

Surprisingly, we now also know that the risk of heart problems is doubled when you have periodontal disease, unless it's controlled. Oral bacteria can aggregate in the mouth, enter the bloodstream, and then attach to plaque developing in your coronary arteries, thus contributing to arterial plaque formation (not just

GLADYS ROJAS DE CHACIN
The limits from diabetes are up to you

A Venezuelan, Gladys Rojas de Chacin has been living with diabetes since she reached the age of fifty over eight years ago. She hasn't let diabetes get her down, though. Her attitude is that diabetes is one of the few illnesses that allow you to take control of your life, and the limits are up to you. She wasn't that surprised when she was diagnosed with diabetes because it was blamed on her obesity, and she accepted it easily and understood the importance of taking care of herself and her diabetes.

Getting by with only two diabetes medications (Glucophage once daily and Amaryl), she focuses on eating a healthy diet that includes diet bread, ham, light yogurt, nuts, fruit, grilled chicken and beef, vegetables, scrambled eggs, and small amounts of rice. She tests her blood sugar twice a day, once before breakfast and then two hours after it.

For Gladys, the most difficult part of her diabetes regimen is exercising regularly. For the Latino community as a whole, she sees additional barriers to good diabetes management. "First of all the lack of education and information about diabetes is a barrier, and it is also hard to find and afford the medications because the Venezuelan government doesn't focus on creating strategies to help the health of the community."

Gladys receives support primarily from her family. As she says, "My son is my best support, helping me with his constant concern about my health and by searching for new information related to diabetes. The Internet has always been a significant support, especially the website called EsTuDiabetes.com." As for who isn't that helpful, Gladys admits, "My husband hasn't been that helpful because he is always buying candy!" Still, she believes that you can live well with diabetes, particularly if you see your doctor regularly (every three months), get your A1c monitored, take medications if you need to for management of your blood lipids, take your prescribed medications, and eat healthy foods on a regular schedule without skipping snacks and meals.

plaque on your teeth). Periodontal disease also increases a potent clotting agent in the bloodstream called fibrinogen, which increases your chances of getting a blood clot that may cause a heart attack or stroke. To cut down on plaque formation and excessive bacteria in your mouth, brush your teeth and tongue at least twice daily and floss once a day. However, toothbrush trauma can cause gum recession, so learn how to brush correctly and always use a soft toothbrush. Visit a periodontist for deep cleaning and scaling below the gum line if your dentist recommends it. And don't smoke. Any type of smoking accelerates the progression of gum disease, along with heart disease.

Preventing pregnancy complications in Latina women

Compared with the rest of the population, Hispanic women give birth at a younger age and have more children, and likely have higher rates of diabetes during pregnancy (both preexisting type 2 and gestational), accompanied by more birth issues like higher death and complication rates. Recently the rate of women with preexisting diabetes (both type 1 and type 2) has more than doubled for women in the twenty to twenty-nine age range and gone up five times for pregnant teenagers. Latino women are one of the minority groups leading the way in this alarming trend.

If you have diabetes before you get pregnant, it is really important for you to seek advice from your health care provider to gain the best possible control of your blood sugar before you conceive. If you don't, you increase your chances for a miscarriage or stillbirth, and your child has a greater chance of birth defects. Offspring of women who have diabetes or are overweight or obese during pregnancy are also more likely to be obese, overweight, or have diabetes in the future.

Keep in mind too, that unless you are well controlled, your baby is likely to be bigger at birth, which increases his or her risk for developing type 2 diabetes at an earlier age, along with potentially making your labor and delivery more complicated. If you have ever given birth to a child weighing more than nine pounds, you likely had gestational diabetes during your pregnancy and will have it again during your next one. For your health and the protection of your future children, be tested for diabetes both before and during your next pregnancy and work hard to keep your blood sugar as close to normal as possible.

Traveling presents its own set of challenges to diabetes care

Although not a long-term health complication, traveling can present some problems and create some short-term health complications. "Always expect the unexpected" should be the diabetic motto for travel. Although you can't avoid the occasional surprise, adequate preparation before you leave can help you avoid undue stress. For instance, you should come prepared with extra supplies, medications, and even extra batteries for your blood glucose meter and any other diabetes-related equipment you may use (like an insulin pump). Some countries require you to have written documents from your doctor stating that you're allowed to carry medicines or supplies, particularly syringes and needles. It's also helpful to bring copies of all of your prescriptions and a list of your medications, including how much you take of each and when (including doses of different forms of insulin).

Carry all of your diabetes-related supplies with you on board the plane (or at least half of them) because placing them in a checked bag that could potentially be lost or delayed is asking for

Diabetes Travel Tips from the U.S.
Transportation Security Administration (TSA)

- When going through the initial TSA screening process, let the screeners know that you have diabetes and will be carrying your supplies with you.
- Clearly identify your insulin and insulin dispensers (e.g., vials, jet injectors, pens, infusers, and preloaded syringes) with a prescription label with your name on it.
- Your other liquid prescription medicines, such as Symlin, Byetta, and glucagon, must also be clearly identified with a prescription label that matches your ID.
- If you have liquids and gels (including cake icing) to treat hypoglycemia in larger than 3-ounce containers, you must declare these items to security checkpoint personnel.
- You may carry on an unlimited number of unused syringes as long as you also have vials of insulin or other injectable medications with you (although used syringes must be in a Sharps disposal or another approved container).
- In addition, you may carry on blood glucose meters and test strips, continuous blood glucose monitors, lancets, alcohol swabs, control solutions, and other blood glucose monitoring supplies.
- You are free to wear your insulin pump (but advise the screeners that you are wearing it) and carry on all of your insulin pump supplies.
- If you would rather have all of your diabetes-related supplies inspected visually rather than have them go through X-ray inspection, you will need to package all of them in a separate bag to be handed to the screeners before you pass through the checkpoint.
- As travel and security guidelines are in a state of flux, check with a travel agent, TSA (866-289-9673), or the American Diabetes Association (800-DIABETES, or www.diabetes.org) to make sure that no new requirements have come into effect that will impact your travel with diabetes supplies.

trouble (particularly nowadays with the heightened security measures and large number of checked bags). If you are going abroad for a long period of time, you may want to send your additional supplies via insured mail to your destination prior to leaving. Keep your insulin with you in the climate-controlled airplane cabin, since checked baggage is exposed to greater temperature extremes than your carry-on items.

Other problems can arise if you have to buy supplies or insulin outside of the United States. American-sold insulins are all U-100 strength, but other countries may sell more dilute U-40 or U-80 varieties, which require different syringes to match these insulins. If you use the wrong syringe, you may end up taking too low a dose when using U-100 syringes with lower-strength insulins. If you travel to certain areas of the world, diabetic supplies may be hard to come by or expensive to get without your usual insurance coverage.

The American Diabetes Association also recommends that you start your trip with at least double the supplies that you think you'll need, carry a quick-acting source of glucose to treat hypoglycemia in flight, bring a snack like a nutrition bar, carry or wear medical identification, and have your physician's contact information available. If feasible, you may also want to have a list of health care professionals at your destination, especially English-speaking or Spanish-speaking ones if you're not fluent in the languages of the countries you're visiting.

CHAPTER 9: *En pocas palabras*

Diabetes can cause you to develop health complications, but most of them are preventable with improvements in your lifestyle and diabetes management. It is helpful to understand more about them, along with which medical treatments are available to slow or prevent eye, kidney, nerve, heart, gum, and other diabetes-related diseases. Latinos can be greatly affected by complications if they fail to prevent them or treat them in the early stages. Your pregnancy can also be complicated by diabetes unless you control your blood sugar. Traveling with diabetes can present its own set of challenges. However, it is possible to live *la vida buena* even if you develop some diabetes-related health complications with proper treatment.

CHAPTER 10

Staying on the Road to Good Health

In this chapter, we discuss common stumbling blocks to controlling diabetes, such as finding excuses to skip your exercise, dietary backsliding around the holidays, illnesses, and more. Remember to be patient. It takes some time to make your lifestyle changes a permanent habit; however, it will happen if you stick with it. Just don't give up trying. The choice is in your own hands. We know that you can and will choose to do it since your health is at stake. *¡No problema!*

The challenges of educating a Latino community

If you're part of a Latino community, you are more likely to trust someone in your group than an outside doctor or other health care provider. Elicit the support of your Latino community leaders and involve them in the planning, delivery, and evaluation of these educational efforts about health and diabetes. Any information that you or others pass on should also be sensitive to different Latino cultures (since sharing the same language doesn't mean that all values are the same), make educational materials available in Spanish that everyone can understand, and take into account differences in income levels. Churches, libraries, and recreational centers (with child care arrangements, if needed) may be appropriate places to hold educational programs in Latino communities.

Empower yourself with knowledge

You're in charge of your own health and diabetes care, so choose to take responsibility for it by becoming your own diabetes advocate. If you don't trust your doctor, consider seeking a second opinion and empower yourself by using any knowledge you have acquired to seek out better ways to control your diabetes. What you don't know about this disease can come back to hurt you in the form of one health problem or another—unless you take action. Encourage people to obtain factual information instead of falling for hearsay and myths. You can help do that by educating yourself first and then helping to inform the rest of your community.

Start by taking more daily steps

Change your daily habits to stay physically active. For motivation, count how many steps you take and then set daily goals for yourself. Reminding yourself to be more active throughout the day really works. Studies have shown that instructing sedentary, overweight women to walk 10,000 steps per day (monitored by a pedometer) is more effective for increasing their daily exercise than asking them to walk thirty minutes most days of the week. Anyone will benefit immensely from taking at least 10,000 steps each day, but taking even 2,000 more steps every day can make the difference between gaining more weight and losing some. (On average, 3,100 to 4,000 pedometer-counted steps are equivalent to thirty minutes of moderate-intensity walking.) Becoming more conscious of how active you are (or are not) during the day may spur you to add in more steps whenever possible.

The most common reason adults give for not exercising on a regular basis is lack of time. So stop thinking of exercise as planned activity and instead try to move more throughout the day. Likely you will be amazed at how much more active you will become and how little time you sacrifice to do it. Any movement you do increases the amount of energy that you expend in a day. In fact, for most people, the majority of their calorie use during the day comes from unstructured activities (discussed in Chapter 5) rather than from a formal exercise plan.

Wearing an inexpensive pedometer is a simple way to motivate and remind yourself to take those steps. Remember, you can add steps throughout the day doing anything you want to, including gardening and other outdoor work, housework and other chores, salsa and other dancing, and many other activities with a Latino flair.

Overcoming some of the other barriers to activity

There are many other barriers to being physically active, such as bad weather that can keep you from walking outdoors. To deal with that, always have a backup plan, such as walking in the mall or doing an alternate activity like an exercise video at home that day (see Chapter 5 for some recommendations). Not everyone has access to the same exercise opportunities or facilities, and your barriers may include unaffordable or inconvenient exercise facilities, no child care, high crime rates in your neighborhood, and fear for your personal safety during outdoor walking or other activities. Even being told to do culturally inappropriate activities can act as a barrier. If you lack confidence in your ability to be physically active (especially if you're overweight) or lack the support and encouragement you need from your immediate family or close friends, that could be a deterrent. Consider including others in neighborhood walks. If self-motivation is your problem, seek out support from others who are more motivated than you are.

Also, it's easy to trick yourself into being more physically active. If you have a sedentary job, get up and walk around the office, building, or block on your breaks, and take the stairs instead of the elevator whenever you can. If you have a sedentary lifestyle, walk to someone else's office or house to deliver a message instead of relying on the phone or email, and park your car at the far end of the parking lot and walk a little extra to get to your destination. Your activities don't have to be done at a high intensity to be effective for diabetes and weight management. For structured exercise, schedule your activity by writing it down on your calendar as you would for other appointments or activities. Doing so makes it more likely that you will actually follow through.

Physical activity will give you more energy, not less

Do you often complain about being too tired to exercise? You may not realize that your lack of exercise is probably responsible for making you feel that way. Even active individuals who take a few weeks off from their normal activities begin to feel sluggish, lethargic, and unmotivated. Start moving more, and you will begin to feel more energized rather than less. When you feel tired, instead of taking a nap, take a short walk and notice how it makes you feel—likely recharged.

Tips for Keeping Your Lifestyle Change Motivation Strong

- Get yourself an exercise buddy (or even a dog that needs to be walked).
- Use sticker charts or other motivational tools to track your progress (for both exercise and dietary changes).
- Schedule structured exercise into your day on your calendar or to-do list.
- Break your larger goals into smaller, realistic stepping-stones (e.g., daily and weekly physical activity goals) for all of your lifestyle changes.
- Reward yourself for meeting your goals with noncaloric treats or outings.
- Plan to do fun physical activities that you really enjoy as often as possible.
- Wear a pedometer (at least occasionally) as a reminder to take more daily steps.
- Have a backup plan that includes alternate activities in case of inclement weather or other barriers to your planned exercise and alternate healthy food choices.
- Distract yourself during exercise by reading a book or magazine, watching TV, listening to music or a book on tape, or talking with a friend.
- Don't start out exercising too intensely or you're likely to get discouraged or injured.
- If you get out of your normal routine and are having trouble getting restarted, simply take small steps in that direction.

Don't let bad health be your excuse for inactivity

Poor health is another major barrier to exercise participation, but not an insurmountable one. Physical activity improves your health in many ways; it is simply a misperception that you can't exercise because of your ailing health. Among the elderly, not just poor health but also age itself may be considered an exercise barrier. We are all aging and losing muscle mass as time marches on, but you can fight the decline by being active. Most of the diseases associated with age are actually caused by a sedentary lifestyle, not advancing age, so most can be reversed to a large extent by being active. For elderly adults, engaging in a functional tasks exercise program may be more effective for maintaining and increasing the ability to perform daily activities than a resistance exercise program. Just remember that resistance exercise definitely helps combat the loss of your muscle mass over time.

Make all of your lifestyle changes more convenient

Another barrier to exercise is that it is inconvenient, especially when no parks, walking trails, fitness centers, or community recreational centers are located nearby. You can alternately engage in home-based programs, which you are more likely to adhere to over the long term than center-based programs because they're more convenient. If you have a seldom-used piece of exercise equipment in your house (or can borrow one from someone), bring it out and start using it regularly. There's so much you can do while working out, like having a conversation in person or on the phone, catching up on your reading, listening to music, or watching your favorite show. Having a distraction will make the time pass quickly. You owe it to yourself and your health to take this time for yourself.

As for your dietary changes, make sure you keep your house and refrigerator well stocked with healthy food choices, such as fresh produce, reduced-fat yogurt, and lean meats. Cut up vegetables and keep them in containers in the refrigerator so that you can pull them out to eat as a quick snack. Don't buy the foods that you're trying to avoid eating. If it's inconvenient to run out and get a high-sugar, high-fat food, you are more likely to eat what you have available instead. Plan your menus ahead of time to avoid relying on quick (and possibly unhealthy) meals, such as microwave pizza, at the last minute. Make meals a family time when you can relax, enjoy each other's company, and share healthy foods and conversation.

Check for fun activities in your community

To become more involved in structured exercise programs, find out what exercise programs are located in your workplace or community. You can often find groups of health-conscious people walking together during lunch breaks, or you may be able to join a low-impact aerobics or other exercise class offered at your workplace or a nearby recreation center. Other activity programs may be available in your area, including formal or informal dance classes through community centers or other recreation-oriented groups. Take the time to find out what is available in your area.

The more you can get involved in making your lifestyle changes as part of a larger community—particularly a Latino one—the more likely you are to be successful in making them a lifelong habit. There's no need to go it alone. Having a regular (and reliable) exercise buddy increases your likelihood of participating, and it also makes your activities more social and fun. Get your spouse, family members, friends, and coworkers to join in your physical activities, especially during your leisure time, as having a good social network to support your exercise habit will help your adherence over the long run. Before having get-togethers that involve food, talk with your guests to see if you can come up with healthier items that everyone can share and enjoy. Across all cultures, ages, and sexes, social support from family, peers, communities, and health care providers results in better motivation and adherence for both dietary and exercise changes.

Finally, your exercise and dietary changes should be as uncomplicated as possible—geared toward your unique health needs, beliefs, and goals—and enjoyable. Most adults need exercise to be fun, or they lose their motivation to do it over time. To prevent boredom with your exercise program, try varying your exercise frequently—both what you do and how hard or long you do it. Knowing that you don't have to do the same workout day after day is motivating. Also, try to pick activities you truly enjoy, such as salsa dancing or golfing (as long as you walk and carry your own clubs). Have fun with your activities to more easily make them a permanent and integral part of your diabetes management. Also, try out new, healthy menus and alternate foods to spice up your diet and keep motivation high.

THAYLU ROJAS
Staying active and upbeat with diabetes and dancing

Teenager Thaylu Rojas of Venezuela has had type 1 diabetes for five years, since the age of nine. To manage her diabetes effectively, she wears an insulin pump that can vary the basal rates for better insulin coverage at different times of day. Her mother, Melissa Cipriani, also tries to keep Thaylu eating a balanced diet (even though she has a sweet tooth). As Melissa recounts, "One of Thaylu's main barriers to good control is getting her to learn portion control and carb counting. She relies on me to count her carbs, but when I'm not around, she seems to overestimate, which often results in hypoglycemia because she gives more insulin than she needs to." The whole family has learned to read food labels to try to help out.

Aside from testing her blood sugar five to six times a day, Thaylu also manages her diabetes by being physically active. She takes dance lessons—tap and jazz—for two hours, twice a week. Because of Thaylu's age, her mother helps manage the pump doses when Thaylu is more active. "As the mother of a diabetic child," Melissa says, "I worry a lot about the future and possible complications related to bad diabetes control. I talk to her and tell her all about the complications of bad control. Sometimes she seems to pay attention, but sometimes she acts as if she doesn't care. I guess that is a part of being a teenager."

In Venezuela there are a lot of misconceptions and a lack of information about diabetes. "When people learn that my daughter has diabetes," Melissa says, "they feel sorry for her as if it's a death sentence. I hear people say that now she can't eat any starches or carbs, and I have to explain to them that she has a balanced diet that consists of all the food groups, which, along with using the correct amount of insulin and doing an exercise routine, gives her good control of her blood sugar." Thaylu's mother is also convinced that the key to living well with diabetes is education and information, which supply the tools needed to make informed decisions. A good diabetes care team is also essential. Melissa reports, "My daughter has a good endocrinologist, nutritionist, ophthalmologist, and pediatrician. We are always reading and researching in order to be informed and educated about diabetes management."

Melissa thinks that her daughter has benefited by having people to look up to who have diabetes as well. "The best thing that has happened to teens with diabetes is Nick Jonas [of the Jonas Brothers singing group]. Since he became public about his condition, my daughter and other teens with diabetes look up to him and the way he so candidly speaks about his having diabetes."

Reward yourself for meeting your goals

Who says that sticker charts and treats are just for kids? Set realistic exercise goals or milestones to keep track of your exercise and dietary changes, and set up rewards for yourself when you meet them. If it works for you, use a sticker chart or some other visible record of physical activities or dietary goals that you accomplish each day and then give yourself frequent reinforcement with tokens or treats (preferably noncaloric ones) when you meet your expectations. Maybe you can promise yourself an outing to somewhere special, the purchase of a coveted item, or anything else that is reasonable and effectively motivates you to exercise. Break up your larger goals into stepping-stone goals, by the day, week, and month, and if you miss one of your goals, try to make the rest of them happen anyway. Making goals open-ended (like saying that you are going to exercise three times a week without trying to schedule the days in advance) often sets you up for failure, so make them more definite. Helpful recommendations for physical activities, activity logs, food journals, and other motivational tools are also widely available.

Be gentle with yourself on your bad days

You will have days when you want to forget you have diabetes or pre-diabetes and chuck your lifestyle changes out the window. Part of making lifelong changes for better health is to learn how to conquer your resistance to change and finding your way back to a healthier way of living—even on the bad days. Think about how much better you felt when you made the changes to motivate yourself. If you find yourself reverting to your old ways, either in minor or major ways, view today as a new day and get back on track. A short break from your routine because of a vacation, illness, or athletic injury does not mean that you can't start scheduling your physical activity back in again or revamp your diet yet again. During any break, be it short or long, try to keep up all of your extra movement during the day even if you can't manage to do anything else to help keep your fitness level higher, which will make it easier to get back into regular exercise as quickly as possible. As soon as possible, move your eating back in the right direction if you've gone off track with that as well.

If you're resuming your exercise after a lapse, remember that you may need to begin at a lower intensity (lighter weights, less re-sistance, or a slower walking speed) of exercise to avoid burnout, muscle soreness, or injury. Even doing only five to ten minutes at a time (instead of thirty or more minutes) is fine. If you really don't want to exercise, make a deal with yourself that you will only do it for a short time to get yourself started (which is often the hardest part). Once you are actually up and moving, you may feel good enough to exceed the time you tricked yourself into doing. The key is to begin through any means possible. As for your diet, try using your blood glucose meter more frequently after a lapse to prove to yourself how great an effect your food choices can have. You may also want to journal how you feel physically; chances are you'll have more energy and feel better overall once you get yourself back to a healthier lifestyle. You're in this for the long term, so even if you're taking small steps in the right direction, you will eventually reach your goals.

Not all bodily changes are related to diabetes

Aging by itself causes bodily changes, many of which have nothing at all to do with diabetes. The aging process involves a gradual decline in the physiological function of your body's systems. Human cells apparently have a limited number of times that they can split and reproduce before dying, and once cells slow their rate of turnover, aging accelerates. The onset of some chronic diseases is often inseparable from aging, but they are not inevitable with advancing age. Even if we could find a way to prevent all disease, hospitals would still be full of people dying of nothing in particular except old age.

Prevention of early death or impairment from treatable problems, though, is an essential part of longevity with and without diabetes. For example, physical activity can offset declining muscle mass (at least to a point) and allow you to retain more of your muscular strength. The diabetes-related benefit is that having more insulin-sensitive muscle mass where glucose can be stored helps to keep your blood sugar under better control. Thus to live long and well, you have to be vigilant about all aspects of your health. Don't hesitate to seek out the doctors and specialists that you need to in order to stay healthy. Never assume that your health will be static. You have to get things treated and see all the necessary physicians—like a cardiologist, an ophthalmologist, and more. You should address your mental health as well, since the stress of diabetes and life in general can affect your care and your sugar control.

If you smoke, get help with stopping

Smoking is one of the worst health habits ever, and when you have diabetes, its effects on your health can be even more dramatic. In general, smokers are more insulin resistant, exhibit several aspects of the insulin resistance syndrome (like elevated blood fats), and have about a 50 percent higher risk of developing type 2 diabetes. If you have type 1, smoking can make you develop double diabetes, or symptoms of both types. It increases your risk of kidney, eye, and nerve problems, as well as heart attack, stroke, and peripheral vascular disease—likely by increasing inflammation around your body and reducing blood flow. Thus smoking cessation is of utmost importance to facilitate control over your blood sugar and to limit the possible development of diabetic complications.

Nicotine in tobacco severely restricts the blood flow to your hands and feet. Since those are the two primary areas of the body afflicted by diabetes-related nerve damage, smoking worsens the potentially devastating effects on your feet and hands. Smoking is also a major, independent risk factor for all types of cardiovascular problems in people without diabetes. And since diabetes itself is a strong risk factor, you're likely more than doubling your risk of having such problems if you smoke. There are many smoking cessation programs, listed at Smoke Free (www.smokefree.gov). Nicotine patches and gum can help lessen your addiction to nicotine. If you still smoke, think long and hard about how healthy you want to be. If your health is a priority, find the help you need to stop or at least cut way back.

CHAPTER 10: *En pocas palabras*
Staying motivated to lead a healthier lifestyle requires effort, but there are things you can do that will help. For instance, empower yourself with knowledge about how to live *la vida buena* with diabetes and share that knowledge with others. Take small steps in the right direction, literally and figuratively, by moving more each day and using a pedometer for motivation. Find ways to overcome barriers to exercise and healthier eating by having backup plans, making lifestyle changes more convenient, making exercise enjoyable, and rewarding yourself for meeting your goals. If you start to backslide into your old habits, start anew on your healthier ones. Finally, if you smoke, find the help you need to stop for better health.

CONCLUSION

Taking on Diabetes . . . and Winning

Given the positive examples of the diabetic Latinos presented throughout the book as well as the abundance of educational tips and advice, if you are part of the Latino community—regardless of the country of origin for you or your relatives—you should walk away from reading this book with the knowledge and confidence to live well with diabetes or prediabetes. Now you know how to follow the path to *la vida buena* with confidence, and you know that it can be done. Now the decision to do so is up to you to turn *¡Qué problema!* into *¡No problema!*

Forget fad diets and stop obsessing over what you eat. Even with small reductions in your weight (such as 5 to 7 percent, or 10 to 15 pounds for most people), which often occur over time as you become more active and make small changes in your dietary patterns, the majority of health benefits will be yours. Lifestyle choices play the biggest role in determining whether you develop obesity, prediabetes, or diabetes, and these conditions can all be improved without dieting.

If your diabetes has not been well controlled up to this point, it's still not too late to start and begin reaping some of the health benefits of improving your control. You may be able to slow the progression of or reverse some of your complications with a little more diligence to your blood sugar. Diabetes care is rapidly changing nowadays, and there are new monitoring tools and medications to better control glycemic peaks and valleys. You should have access to everything that you need to manage your diabetes effectively.

The following list summarizes the key behaviors for living long and well with diabetes or prediabetes:

- Regularly monitor your blood glucose levels.
- Watch your diet and make healthier food choices by eating less refined foods naturally rich in antioxidants, vitamins and minerals, and fiber.
- Exercise and stay as physically active as possible on a daily basis.
- Set goals, particularly ones that focus on good health habits.
- Learn all you can about diabetes and how to control it and avoid complications.
- Involve a supportive spouse, family, or friends—including maybe your greater Latino community—in your diabetes care.
- Maintain a positive attitude about diabetes and life in general.
- Share your diabetes knowledge with others.
- Find a good doctor, preferably an endocrinologist, or a diabetes educator that you trust who can help you better manage your condition.
- Always take your insulin or other prescribed medications to control your blood sugar.

If you do all these things, your health will benefit and your body will be as healthy as possible. Remember, it's never too late to get started on a path to a healthier, more vital you. Dr. Sheri and Dr. Leo *te deseamos lo mejor y sabemos que tú puedes*. Get started today!

APPENDIX A

Important Websites for Diabetic (and Prediabetic) Latinos

American Association of Diabetes Educators (diabetes information and educator locator): www.diabeteseducator.org
   Diabetes educator locator: www.diabeteseducator.org/DiabetesEducation/Find.html
   American College of Sports Medicine: www.acsm.org
   Exercise Is Medicine public health campaign: www.exerciseismedicine.org
   American Council on Exercise (ACE) (health and fitness tips, fitness Q&A): www.acefitness.org/fitfacts
American Diabetes Association (ADA) (diabetes information, links, bookstore): www.diabetes.org
   Carb counting: www.diabetes.org/for-parents-and-kids/diabetes-care/carb-count.jsp
   Club Ped: www.diabetes.org/ClubPed/index.jsp (pedometer walking club)
   Diabetes information en Español: www.diabetes.org/espanol/default.jsp
   Latino health care information: www.diabetes.org/for-health-professionals-and-scientists/latino-health-care.jsp
American Dietetic Association (nutrition information for consumers): www.eatright.org/Public
American Obesity Association (obesity information, advocacy, and statistics): www.obesity.org
America on the Move (national initiative to improve health and quality of life): www.americaonthemove.org

223

Argentina Diabetes Society (Sociedad Argentina de Diabetes): www.diabetes
.org.ar

Calories per Hour (physical activity and metabolic calculators and information): www.caloriesperhour.com

Center for Nutrition Policy and Promotion (CNPP) (nutrition policy, healthy
eating index): www.cnpp.usda.gov

Interactive Healthy Eating Index and Physical Activity Tool: http://147.208
.9.133

Center for Science in the Public Interest (Nutrition Action newsletter and
other information): www.cspinet.org

Centers for Disease Control and Prevention (CDC) (U.S. government agency):
www.cdc.gov/health/diabetes.htm

Overweight and obesity facts: www.cdc.gov/nccdphp/dnpa/obesity/index.htm

Chef LaLa (TV celebrity and certified nutritionist specializing in light Latino
recipes): www.cheflala.com

Diabetes Exercise and Sports Association (DESA) (activity-related diabetes
organization): www.diabetes-exercise.org

Diabetes Health magazine (research updates, educational articles, product
guides): www.diabeteshealth.com

Diabetes in Control (weekly diabetes research updates): www.diabetesincontrol
.com

Diabetes Juvenil (type 1 diabetes information in Spanish): www.diabetesjuvenil
.com

Diabetes Mine (diabetes-related blog by Amy Tenderich): www.diabetesmine.com

Diabetes Sports and Wellness Foundation: www.dswf.org

Diabetic Connect (diabetes community, articles, and blogs): www.diabetic
connect.com

Disabled Sports USA (sports information for people with disabilities, including vision loss): www.dsusa.org

dLife—For Your Diabetes Life (multimedia diabetes information, advocacy,
and interaction): www.dlife.com

Recipe database (with food look-up option): www.dlife.com/diabetic-
recipes.html

Eating Well: The Magazine of Food and Health (nutrition articles and healthy
recipes): www.eatingwell.com/index.htm

Es Tu Diabetes (Spanish version of social network for diabetic Latinos): www
.estudiabetes.com

Glycemic Index Information and Database (glycemic index information): www
.glycemicindex.com

Hispanopolis (health and other programming in Spanish): www.hispanopolis
.com

IDEA Health and Fitness Association (fitness articles and personal trainer locator service): www.ideafit.com

Insulite Laboratories (diabetes, prediabetes, and weight management proto-
cols): www.insulitelabs.com

Joslin Diabetes Center (prominent diabetes treatment center in Boston, nutrition guidelines): www.joslin.org
    Nutritional guidelines for type 2s: www.joslin.org/Files/Nutrition_ClinGuide
        .pdf

Just Move.Org (fitness center, progress tracker by the American Heart Association): www.justmove.org

Juvenile Diabetes Research Foundation: www.jdrf.org

Latino Nutrition Coalition (nutrition and other health-related information for
Latinos): www.latinonutrition.org

Latinos In Shape (nutrition and health articles in Spanish): www.latinosin
shape.com

Lifelong Exercise Institute (exercise assistance and programming): www.life
longexercise.com

Mexican Federation of Diabetes (Federación Mexicana de Diabetes): www.fm
diabetes.org

National Center on Physical Activity and Disability (NCPAD) (lifetime sports
with disabilities): www.ncpad.org

National Diabetes Education Program: www.ndep.nih.gov/index.htm
    Minority campaigns: www.ndep.nih.gov/campaigns/campaigns_index.htm
    Prevengamos la Diabetes Tipo 2, Paso a Paso: www.ndep.nih.gov/campaigns/
        Tipo2/Tipo2_index.htm

National Institutes of Health (NIH) (U.S. government health agency): www
.nih.gov
    Body mass index (BMI) calculator: www.nhlbisupport.com/bmi/bmicalc.htm
    Facts about dietary supplements: www.cc.nih.gov/ccc/supplements
    Interactive menu planner: www.hp2010.nhlbihin.net/menuplanner/menu.cgi
    Senior health information (all topics): http://nihseniorhealth.gov

National Sports Center for the Disabled (NSCD) (sports events information
for disabled persons): www.nscd.org

National Weight Control Registry (successful weight loss registry and information): www.nwcr.ws

Nutridiary (free online food and exercise diary, food nutrient database): www
.nutridiary.com

Nutrition Data (nutrition data by food item, nutrient density, calorie counter): www.nutritiondata.com

Nutritional Analysis Tool (NATS 2.0) (online food and diet analysis): www .nat.uiuc.edu/mainnat.html

Reflective Happiness (free happiness index, depression scale, and signature strengths surveys): www.reflectivehappiness.com

Shape Up America! (nonprofit group dedicated to achieving a healthy weight for life): www.shapeup.org

Sheri Colberg's website (links to diabetes books, exercise articles, interviews, blog, and more): www.shericolberg.com

Smoke Free (assistance with smoking cessation): www.smokefree.gov

Taking Control of Your Diabetes (nonprofit seminars and diabetes information): www.tcoyd.org

Latino initiative (in Spanish): www.tcoyd.org/SPANISH_INDEX.php

The Diabetes Mall (diabetes supplies and helpful information on pumps, gadgets, and more): www.diabetesnet.com

Carb counting information: www.diabetesnet.com/diabetes_food_diet/carb_ counting.php

The President's Challenge (U.S. government physical activity and fitness awards program): www.presidentschallenge.org

The President's Council on Physical Fitness and Sports (U.S. government fitness council): www.fitness.gov

Tu Diabetes (social network for people with diabetes, particularly Hispanics): www.tudiabetes.com

U.S. Department of Agriculture (USDA) (food guide pyramid, food databases): www.nal.usda.gov/fnic/foodcomp/srch/search.htm

New food guide pyramid: www.mypyramid.gov

U.S. Food and Drug Administration (FDA) (medications and supplement regulatory agency): www.cfsan.fda.gov/~dms/supplmnt.html

Mercury levels in fish: www.cfsan.fda.gov/~dms/admehg3.html

Publications en Español: www.fda.gov/oc/spanish

Weight Control Information Network (WIN) (NIH-provided science-based information on weight control, obesity, physical activity, and related nutritional issues): http://win.niddk.nih.gov/index.htm

APPENDIX B

Glycemic Index (per 50 grams of available carbohydrate) and Glycemic Load (per "typical" serving) (GI, GL) of Common Foods

	Low-GI (0 to 55)	Medium-GI (56 to 69)	High-GI (70 to 100)
Low GL (< 10)	Apples (38,6)	Apricots (57,5)	Bread, white flour (70,10)
	Beans, garbanzo (28,8)	Beets (64,5)	Bread, whole-wheat (71,9)
	Beans, baked (48,7)	Bread, 7-grain (55,8)	Glucose (99,10)
	Beans, butter (33,1)	Cantaloupe (65,4)	Popcorn (72,8)
	Beans, kidney (28,7)	Honey (55,10)	Watermelon (72,4)
	Beans, navy (31,6)	Ice cream, regular (61,8)	
	Beans, pinto (39,10)	Jam, strawberry (51,10)	
	Bread, whole-grain (51,7)	Peaches, canned in heavy syrup (55,9)	
	Carrots, raw (47,3)	Pineapple (59,7)	
	Cereal, All-Bran (42,9)	Sugar, white (68,7)	
	Chickpeas (28,8)		
	Cookie, oatmeal (54,9)		
	Corn, sweet (54,9)		
	Fructose sweetener (20,2)		
	Grapefruit (25,3)		
	Grapes (46,8)		
	Ice cream, low-fat (43,5)		
	Ice cream, premium (38,4)		
	Juice, carrot (43,10)		
	Juice, tomato (38,4)		
	Lentils, red (26,5)		
	M&Ms, peanut (33,6)		
	Milk, skim (32,4)		
	Milk, soy (42,7)		
	Milk, whole (40,3)		
	Oranges (42,5)		
	Peaches (42,5)		
	Peaches, canned in juice (38,9)		
	Peanuts (14,1)		
	Pears (38,4)		
	Peas, green (48,3)		
	Prunes (29,10)		
	Strawberries (40,1)		
	Tortellini, cheese (50,10)		
	Yogurt, low-fat (27,7)		
	Yogurt, nonfat, artificially sweetened (24,3)		

	Low-GI (0 to 55)	Medium-GI (56 to 69)	High-GI (70 to 100)
Medium GL *(11 to 19)*	Bananas (52,12) Barley, pearled (25,11) Beans, navy (38,12) Bread, sourdough wheat (54,15) Buckwheat (54,16) Cookie bar, Twix (44,17) Juice, apple (40,12) Juice, grapefruit (48,11) Juice, orange (50,12) Juice, pineapple (46,16) Pasta, fettuccine (40,18) Ravioli, meat (39,15) Rice, parboiled (47,17)	Cake, angel food (67,19) Cereal, Life (66,16) Cereal, Raisin Bran (61,12) Cereal, Special K (69,14) Croissant (67,17) Juice, orange (57,15) Muffin, bran (60,15) Oatmeal, old-fashioned (58,13) Oatmeal, quick (66,17) Pizza, cheese (60,16) Potatoes, new (57,12) Potatoes, sweet (61,17) Rice, brown, boiled (55,18) Rice, wild (57,18)	Cereal, Cheerios (74,15) Cereal, Grape Nuts (75,16) Cereal, shredded wheat (75,15) Cereal, Total (76,17) Crackers, soda (74,12) Doughnut, cake-type (76,17) Gatorade, 12 oz. (78,17) Muffin, English (77,11) Potatoes, mashed (85,17) Pretzels (83,16) Rice cakes, puffed (78, 17) Wafers, vanilla (77,14)
High GL *(> 20)*	Pasta, linguine (46,22) Pasta, macaroni (47,23) Pasta, spaghetti (44,21)	Candy bar, Mars (65,26) Candy bar, Snickers (68,23) Coca-Cola, 12 oz. can (63,23) Couscous (65,23) Cranberry juice cocktail (68,24) Kudos, whole-grain bar, chocolate chip (62,20) Macaroni and cheese, boxed (64,32) Power Bar (56,24) Raisins (64,28) Rice, white, boiled (64,23)	Bagel, white flour (72,25) Candy, Skittles (70,32) Cereal, cornflakes (92,24) Cereal, Golden Grahams (71,18) Cereal, Crispix (87,22) Cereal, Rice Krispies (82,22) French fries (75,22) Fruit bars, strawberry (90,23) Fruit roll-ups (99,24) Jelly beans (78,22) Pop Tart, double chocolate (70,24) Potato, baked russet (85,26)

SUGGESTED READING

Barnes, Darryl. *Action Plan for Diabetes: Your Guide to Controlling Blood Sugar.* Champaign, IL: Human Kinetics, 2004.

Becker, Gretchen. *The First Year—Type 2 Diabetes: An Essential Guide for the Newly Diagnosed.* New York: Marlowe, 2001.

Brand-Miller, Jennie, et al. *The New Glucose Revolution.* New York: Marlowe, 2003.

Chef LaLa. *Latin Lover Lite.* Agoura Hills, CA: Spencer, 2004.

Colberg, Sheri R. *Diabetes-Free Kids: A Take-Charge Plan for Preventing and Treating Type 2 Diabetes in Children.* New York: Avery, 2005.

Colberg, Sheri R. *Diabetic Athlete's Handbook: Your Guide to Peak Performance.* Champaign, IL: Human Kinetics, 2008.

Colberg, Sheri R. *The 7 Step Diabetes Fitness Plan: Living Well and Being Fit with Diabetes, No Matter Your Weight.* New York: Marlowe, 2006.

Colberg, Sheri R., and Steven V. Edelman. *50 Secrets of the Longest Living People with Diabetes.* New York: Da Capo Press, 2007.

Diaz-Brown, Laura. *Chef LaLa Presents Best-Loved Mexican Cooking.* Lincolnwood, IL: Publications International, 2008.

Drago, Lorena. *Beyond Beans and Rice (Algo Mas que Arroz con Frijoles).* New York: McGraw-Hill, 2006.

Gaesser, Glenn. *Big Fat Lies: The Truth About Your Weight and Your Health.* Carlsbad, CA: Gürze, 2002.

Hayes, Charlotte. *The "I Hate to Exercise" Book for People with Diabetes.* 2nd ed. Alexandria, VA: American Diabetes Association, 2006.

Hoover, Matt, and Sheri R. Colberg. *Matt Hoover's Guide to Life, Love, and Losing Weight.* New York: Skyhorse, 2008.

Jackson, Richard, and Amy Tenderich. *Know Your Numbers, Outlive Your Diabetes: 5 Essential Health Factors You Can Master to Enjoy a Long and Healthy Life.* New York: Da Capo Press, 2006.

Joseph, James, Daniel Nadeau, and Anne Underwood. *The Color Code: A Revolutionary Eating Plan for Optimal Health.* New York: Hyperion, 2003.

Morley, John E., and Sheri R. Colberg. *The Science of Staying Young.* New York: McGraw-Hill, 2007.

Nathan, David, and Linda Delahanty. *Beating Diabetes.* New York: McGraw-Hill, 2005.

Neporent, Liz, Suzanne Schlosberg, and Shirley Archer. *Weight Training for Dummies.* New York: For Dummies, 2006.

Peters, Anne. *Conquering Diabetes: A Cutting-Edge, Comprehensive Program for Prevention and Treatment.* New York: Hudson Street Press, 2005.

Price, Joan. *The Anytime, Anywhere Exercise Book.* Avon, MA: Adams Media Corporation, 2003.

Scheiner, Gary. *Think Like a Pancreas: A Practical Guide to Managing Diabetes with Insulin.* New York: Marlowe, 2004.

Scheiner, Gary. *The Ultimate Guide to Accurate Carb Counting: Featuring the Tools and Techniques Used by the Experts.* New York: Da Capo Press, 2006.

Warshaw, Hope S. *Eat Out, Eat Right: A Guide to Healthier Restaurant Eating.* Chicago: Agate Surrey, 2008.

SELECTED REFERENCES

Introduction: Why Latinos Need to Take on the Diabetes Problema *Now*

American Association of Diabetes Educators. 2002. Intensive diabetes management: Implications of the DCCT and UKPDS. *Diabetes Educator* 28:735–740.

Goldberg, R. B. 2003. Cardiovascular disease in patients who have diabetes. *Cardiology Clinics* 21:399–413.

Narayan, K., J. Boyle, T. Thompson et al. 2003. Lifetime risk for diabetes mellitus in the United States. *Journal of the American Medical Association* 290:1884–1890.

National Diabetes Information Clearinghouse. National Diabetes Statistics, 2007. Accessed at http://diabetes.niddk.nih.gov/dm/pubs/statistics/#allages.

Smith, C. A., E. Barnett. 2005. Diabetes-related mortality among Mexican Americans, Puerto Ricans, and Cuban Americans in the United States. *Pan American Journal of Public Health* 18:381–387.

Sullivan, P. W., E. H. Morrato, V. Ghushchyan et al. 2005. Obesity, inactivity, and the prevalence of diabetes and diabetes-related cardiovascular comorbidities in the U.S., 2000–2002. *Diabetes Care* 28:1599–1603.

Chapter 1: Living La Vida Buena *with Diabetes in a Latino Culture*

Aas, A. M., I. Bergstad, P. M. Thorsby et al. 2005. An intensified lifestyle intervention programme may be superior to insulin treatment in poorly controlled type 2 diabetic patients on oral hypoglycaemic agents: Results of a feasibility study. *Diabetic Medicine* 22:316–322.

Ciechanowski, P. S., W. J. Katon, J. E. Russo, E. A. Walker. 2001. The patient-provider relationship: Attachment theory and adherence to treatment in diabetes. *American Journal of Psychiatry* 158:29–35.

Franciosi, M., F. Pellegrini, G. De Berardis et al. 2001. The impact of blood glucose self-monitoring on metabolic control and quality of life in type 2 diabetic patients: An urgent need for better educational strategies. *Diabetes Care* 24:1870–1877.

Lerman, I., L. Lozano, A. R. Villa et al. 2004. Psychosocial factors associated with poor diabetes self-care management in a specialized center in Mexico City. *Biomedicine and Pharmacotherapy* 58:566–570.

Millan-Ferro, A., A. E. Caballero. 2007. Cultural approaches to diabetes self-management programs for the Latino community. *Current Diabetes Reports* 7:391–397.

Murata, G. H., J. H. Shah, R. M. Hoffman et al. 2003. Intensified blood glucose monitoring improves glycemic control in stable, insulin-treated veterans with type 2 diabetes: The Diabetes Outcomes in Veterans Study (DOVES). *Diabetes Care* 26:1759–1763.

Nguyen, T. T., N. A. Daniels, G. L. Gildengorin, E. J. Perez-Stable. 2007. Ethnicity, language, specialty care, and quality of diabetes care. *Ethnicity & Disease* 17:65–71.

Rafique, G., F. Shaikh. 2006. Identifying needs and barriers to diabetes education in patients with diabetes. *Journal of the Pakistan Medical Association* 56:347–352.

Schalch, A., J. Ybarra, D. Adler et al. 2001. Evaluation of a psycho-educational nutritional program in diabetic patients. *Patient Education and Counseling* 44:171–178.

Tankova, T., G. Dakovska, D. Koev. 2004. Education and quality of life in diabetic patients. *Patient Education and Counseling* 53:285–290.

Chapter 2: Understanding Body Fat, Fitness, and Diabetes

Bellisle, F., A. M. Dalix, M. A. De Assis et al. 2007. Motivational effects of 12-week moderately restrictive diets with or without special attention to the glycaemic index of foods. *British Journal of Nutrition* 97:790–798.

Biddinger, S. B., A. Hernandez-Ono, C. Rask-Madsen et al. 2008. Hepatic insulin resistance is sufficient to produce dyslipidemia and susceptibility to atherosclerosis. *Cell Metabolism* 7:125–134.

Brooks, N., J. E. Layne, P. L. Gordon et al. 2006. Strength training improves muscle quality and insulin sensitivity in Hispanic older adults with type 2 diabetes. *International Journal of Medical Sciences* 4:19–27.

Caballero, A. E., K. Bousquet-Santos, L. Robles-Osorio et al. 2008. Overweight Latino children and adolescents have marked endothelial dysfunction and subclinical vascular inflammation in association with excess body fat and insulin resistance. *Diabetes Care* 31:576–582.

Clark, M. 2004. Is weight loss a realistic goal of treatment in type 2 diabetes? The implications of restraint theory. *Patient Counseling and Education* 53:277–283.

Cruz, M. L., M. J. Weigensberg, T. T. Huang et al. 2004. The metabolic syndrome in overweight Hispanic youth and the role of insulin sensitivity. *Journal of Clinical Endocrinology and Metabolism* 89:108–113.

Diaz, V. A., A. G. Mainous 3rd, C. Pope. 2007. Cultural conflicts in the weight loss experience of overweight Latinos. *International Journal of Obesity* 31:328–333.

Farshchi, H. R., M. A. Taylor, I. A. Macdonald. 2005. Deleterious effects of omitting breakfast on insulin sensitivity and fasting lipid profiles in healthy lean women. *American Journal of Clinical Nutrition* 81:388–396.

Field, A. E., S. B. Austin, C. B. Taylor et al. 2003. Relation between dieting and weight change among preadolescents and adolescents. *Pediatrics* 112:900–906.

Hamman, R. F., R. R. Wing, S. L. Edelstein et al. 2006. Effect of weight loss with lifestyle intervention on risk of diabetes. *Diabetes Care* 29:2102–2107.

Hu, F. B., R. J. Sigal, J. W. Rich-Edwards et al. 1999. Walking compared with vigorous physical activity and risk of type 2 diabetes in women: A prospective study. *Journal of the American Medical Association* 282:1433–1439.

Jebb, S. A. 2005. Dietary strategies for the prevention of obesity. *Proceedings of the Nutrition Society* 64:217–227.

Kadoglou, N. P., F. Iliadis, N. Angelopoulou et al. 2007. The anti-inflammatory effects of exercise training in patients with type 2 diabetes mellitus. *European Journal of Cardiovascular Prevention and Rehabilitation* 14:637–643.

Kruger, J., H. M. Blanck, C. Gillespie. 2006. Dietary and physical activity behaviors among adults successful at weight loss maintenance. *International Journal of Behavioral Nutrition and Physical Activity* 3:17.

Lane, J. D., M. N. Feinglos, R. S. Surwit. 2008. Caffeine increases ambulatory glucose and postprandial responses in coffee drinkers with type 2 diabetes. *Diabetes Care* 31:221–222.

Lane, J. D., A. L. Hwang, M. N. Feinglos, R. S. Surwit. 2007. Exaggeration of postprandial hyperglycemia in patients with type 2 diabetes by administration of caffeine in coffee. *Endocrinology Practice* 13:239–243.

Leser, M. S., S. Z. Yanovski, J. A. Yanovski. 2002. A low-fat intake and greater activity level are associated with lower weight regain 3 years after completing a very-low-calorie diet. *Journal of the American Dietetics Association* 102:1252–1256.

Li, G., P. Zhang, J. Wang et al. 2008. The long-term effect of lifestyle interventions to prevent diabetes in the China Da Qing Diabetes Prevention Study: A 20-year follow-up study. *Lancet* 371:1783–1789.

Lindström, J., P. Ilanne-Parikka, M. Peltonen et al. 2006. Sustained reduction in the incidence of type 2 diabetes by lifestyle intervention: Follow-up of the Finnish Diabetes Prevention Study. *Lancet* 368:1673–1679.

Lindström, J., M. Peltonen, J. G. Eriksson et al. 2006. High-fibre, low-fat diet predicts long-term weight loss and decreased type 2 diabetes risk: The Finnish Diabetes Prevention Study. *Diabetologia* 49:912–920.

Mayers, D. 2005. Is dieting bad for you? Experts debate whether losing weight is the wrong prescription for better health. *Diabetes Health* 14:50–52, 54–55.

Nagano, M., Y. Kai, B. Zou et al. 2004. The contribution of cardiorespiratory fitness and visceral fat to risk factors in Japanese patients with impaired glucose tolerance and type 2 diabetes mellitus. *Metabolism* 53:644–649.

Raynor, H. A., R. W. Jeffery, S. Phelan et al. 2005. Amount of food group variety consumed in the diet and long-term weight loss maintenance. *Obesity Research* 13:883–890.

Rodearmel, S. J., H. R. Wyatt, N. Stroebele et al. 2007. Small changes in dietary sugar and physical activity as an approach to preventing excessive weight gain: The America on the Move family study. *Pediatrics* 120:e869–e879.

Solomon, T. P., S. N. Sistrun, R. K. Krishnan et al. 2008. Exercise and diet enhance fat oxidation and reduce insulin resistance in older obese adults. *Journal of Applied Physiology* 104:1313–1319.

Stevens, J., J. Cai, K. Evenson, R. Thomas. 2002. Fitness and fatness as predictors of mortality from all causes and from cardiovascular disease in men and women in the Lipid Research Clinics Study. *American Journal of Epidemiology* 156:832–841.

Sui, X., S. P. Hooker, I. M. Lee et al. 2008. A prospective study of cardiorespiratory fitness and risk of type 2 diabetes in women. *Diabetes Care* 31:550–555.

Sui, X., M. J. LaMonte, J. N. Laditka et al. 2007. Cardiorespiratory fitness and adiposity as mortality predictors in older adults. *Journal of the American Medical Association* 298:2507–2516.

Vogels, N., M. S. Westerterp-Plantenga. Successful long-term weight maintenance: A 2-year follow-up. *Obesity* 15:1258–1266.

Wadden, T. A., M. L. Butryn, K. J. Byrne. 2004. Efficacy of lifestyle modification for long-term weight control. *Obesity Research* 12:151S–162S.

Wang, M. Y., P. Grayburn, S. Chen et al. 2008. Adipogenic capacity and the susceptibility to type 2 diabetes and metabolic syndrome. *Proceedings of the National Academy of Sciences of the United States of America* 105:6139–6144.

Wang, Y., E. B. Rimm, M. J. Stampfer et al. 2005. Comparison of abdominal adiposity and overall obesity in predicting risk of type 2 diabetes among men. *American Journal of Clinical Nutrition* 81:555–563.

Wing, R., J. Hill. 2001. Successful weight loss maintenance. *Annual Reviews in Nutrition* 21:323–341.

Whitmer, R. A., E. P. Gunderson, E. Barrett-Connor et al. 2005. Obesity in middle age and future risk of dementia: A 27-year longitudinal population-based study. *British Medical Journal* 330:1360–1364.

Chapter 3: Going Beyond the Latino Diet

American Diabetes Association. 2008. Clinical practice recommendations: Nutrition recommendations and interventions for diabetes. *Diabetes Care* 31:S61–S78.

Arora, S. K., S. I. McFarlane. 2005. The case for low carbohydrate diets in diabetes management. *Nutrition & Metabolism* (Lond) 2:16.

Bazzano, L. A., T. Y. Li, K. J. Joshipura, F. B. Hu. 2008. Intake of fruit, vegetables, and fruit juices and risk of diabetes in women. *Diabetes Care* 31:1311–1317.

Boden, G., K. Sargrad, C. Homko et al. 2005. Effect of a low-carbohydrate diet on appetite, blood glucose levels, and insulin resistance in obese patients with type 2 diabetes. *Annals of Internal Medicine* 142:403–411.

Brand-Miller, J., S. Hayne, P. Petocz, S. Colagiuri. 2003. Low-glycemic index diets in the management of diabetes: A meta-analysis of randomized control trials. *Diabetes Care* 26:2261–2267.

Burani, J., P. J. Longo. 2006. Low-glycemic index carbohydrates: An effective behavioral change for glycemic control and weight management in patients with type 1 and 2 diabetes. *Diabetes Educator* 32:78–88.

Chiu, K., A. Chu, V. Go, M. Saad. 2004. Low vitamin D worsens beta cell function. *American Journal of Clinical Nutrition* 79:820–825.

Ebbeling, C. B., M. M. Leidig, K. B. Sinclair et al. 2003. A reduced-glycemic load diet in the treatment of adolescent obesity. *Archives of Pediatric and Adolescent Medicine* 157:773–779.

Foster-Powell, K., S. Holt, J. Brand-Miller. 2002. International table of glycemic index and glycemic load values, 2002. *American Journal of Clinical Nutrition* 76:5–56.

Galgani, J., C. Aguirre, E. Diaz. 2006. Acute effect of meal glycemic index and glycemic load on blood glucose and insulin responses in humans. *Nutrition Journal* 5:22.

Goudswaard, A., R. Stalk, H. de Valk, G. Rutten. 2003. Improving glycaemic control in patients with type 2 diabetes mellitus without insulin therapy. *Diabetic Medicine* 20:540–544.

Grassi, D., C. Lippi, S. Necozione et al. 2005. Short-term administration of dark chocolate is followed by a significant increase in insulin sensitivity and a decrease in blood pressure in healthy persons. *American Journal of Clinical Nutrition* 81:611–614.

Hess-Fischl, A. 2007. Beyond rice and beans: The Caribbean Latino guide to eating healthy with diabetes. *Diabetes Educator* 33:460–462.

Jayaprakasam, B., S. K. Vareed, L. K. Olson et al. 2005. Insulin secretion by bioactive anthocyanins and anthocyanidins present in fruits. *Journal of Agricultural and Food Chemistry* 53:28–31.

Koppes, L. L., J. M. Dekker, H. F. Hendriks et al. 2005. Moderate alcohol consumption lowers the risk of type 2 diabetes: A meta-analysis of prospective observational studies. *Diabetes Care* 28:719–725.

Lane, J. D., M. N. Feinglos, R. S. Surwit. 2008. Caffeine increases ambulatory glucose and postprandial responses in coffee drinkers with type 2 diabetes. *Diabetes Care* 31:221–222.

Lane, J. D., A. L. Hwang, M. N. Feinglos, R. S. Surwit. 2007. Exaggeration of postprandial hyperglycemia in patients with type 2 diabetes by administration of caffeine in coffee. *Endocrinology Practice* 13:239–243.

Lee, S., R. Hudson, K. Kilpatrick et al. 2005. Caffeine ingestion is associated with reductions in glucose uptake independent of obesity and type 2 diabetes before and after exercise training. *Diabetes Care* 28:566–572.

Liu, R. 2003. Health benefits of fruit and vegetables are from additive and synergistic combinations of phytochemicals. *American Journal of Clinical Nutrition* 78:517S–520S.

Lovejoy, J. 2002. The influence of dietary fat on insulin resistance. *Current Diabetes Reports* 2:435–440.

Ma, Y., B. Olendzki, D. Chiriboga et al. 2005. Association between dietary carbohydrates and body weight. *American Journal of Epidemiology* 161:359–367.

O'Keefe, J. H., N. M. Gheewala, J. O. O'Keefe. 2008. Dietary strategies for improving post-prandial glucose, lipids, inflammation, and cardiovascular health. *Journal of the American College of Cardiology* 51:249–255.

Qi, L., E. Rimm, S. Liu et al. 2005. Dietary glycemic index, glycemic load, cereal fiber, and plasma adiponectin concentration in diabetic men. *Diabetes Care* 28:1022–1028.

Rizkalla, S., L. Taghrid, M. Laromiguiere et al. 2004. Improved plasma glucose control, whole-body glucose utilization, and lipid profile on a low-glycemic index diet in type 2 diabetic men. *Diabetes Care* 27:1866–1872.

Sargrad, K. R., C. Homko, M. Mozzoli, G. Boden. 2005. Effect of high protein vs. high carbohydrate intake on insulin sensitivity, body weight, hemoglobin A1c, and blood pressure in patients with type 2 diabetes mellitus. *Journal of the American Dietetic Association* 105:573–580.

Slama, G., F. Elgrably, M. Kabir, S. Rizkalla. 2006. Low glycemic index foods should play a role in improving overall glycemic control in type-1 and type-2 diabetic patients and, more specifically, in correcting excessive postprandial hyperglycemia. Nestlé Nutrition Workshop Series. *Clinical and Performance Program* 11:73–81.

Sugiura, M., M. Nakamura, Y. Ikoma et al. 2006. The homeostasis model assessment-insulin resistance index is inversely associated with serum carotenoids in non-diabetic subjects. *Journal of Epidemiology* 16:71–78.

Willett, W., J. Manson, S. Liu. 2002. Glycemic index, glycemic load, and risk of type 2 diabetes. *American Journal of Clinical Nutrition* 76:274S–280S.

Young, L. R., M. Nestle. 2003. Expanding portion sizes in the US marketplace: Implications for nutrition counseling. *Journal of the American Dietetics Association* 103:231–234.

Zemel, M. B., J. Richards, S. Mathis et al. 2005. Dairy augmentation of total and central fat loss in obese subjects. *International Journal of Obesity* 29:391–397.

Chapter 4: Choosing Supplements Wisely

Albarracin, C. A., B. C. Fuqua, J. L. Evans, and I. D. Goldfine. 2008. Chromium picolinate and biotin combination improves glucose metabolism in treated, uncontrolled overweight to obese patients with type 2 diabetes. *Diabetes/ Metabolism Research and Reviews* 24:41–51.

Albarracin, C., B. Fuqua, J. Geohas et al. 2007. Combination of chromium and biotin improves coronary risk factors in hypercholesterolemic type 2 diabetes mellitus: A placebo-controlled, double-blind randomized clinical trial. *Journal of the Cardiometabolic Syndrome* 2:91–97.

Brazionis, L., K. Rowley, C. Itsiopoulos, K. O'Dea. 2008. Plasma carotenoids and diabetic retinopathy. *British Journal of Nutrition* 13:1–8.

Chausmer, A. 1998. Zinc, insulin, and diabetes. *Journal of the American College of Nutrition* 17:109–115.

Cheng, H. H., M. H. Lai, W. C. Hou, C. L. Huang. 2004. Antioxidant effects of chromium supplementation with type 2 diabetes mellitus and euglycemic subjects. *Journal of Agricultural and Food Chemistry* 52:1385–1389.

Chiu, K., A. Chu, V. Go, M. Saad. 2004. Low vitamin D worsens beta cell function. *American Journal of Clinical Nutrition* 79:820–825.

Cusi, K., S. Cukier, R. DeFronzo et al. 2001. Vanadyl sulfate improves hepatic and muscle insulin sensitivity in type 2 diabetes. *Journal of Clinical Endocrinology and Metabolism* 86:1410–1417.

Eddy, J. J. 2005. Topical honey for diabetic foot ulcers. *Journal of Family Practice* 54:533–535.

Grassi, D., C. Lippi, S. Necozione et al. 2005. Short-term administration of dark chocolate is followed by a significant increase in insulin sensitivity and a decrease in blood pressure in healthy persons. *American Journal of Clinical Nutrition* 81:611–614.

Head, K. A. 2006. Peripheral neuropathy: Pathogenic mechanisms and alternative therapies. *Alternative Medicine Review* 11:294–329.

Hilpert, K. F., S. G. West, P. M. Kris-Etherton et al. 2007. Postprandial effect of n-3 polyunsaturated fatty acids on apolipoprotein B-containing lipoproteins and vascular reactivity in type 2 diabetes. *American Journal of Clinical Nutrition* 85:369–376.

Jayaprakasam, B., S. K. Vareed, L. K. Olson et al. 2005. Insulin secretion by bioactive anthocyanins and anthocyanidins present in fruits. *Journal of Agricultural and Food Chemistry* 53:28–31.

Khan, A., M. Safdar, M. M. Ali Khan et al. 2003. Cinnamon improves glucose and lipids of people with type 2 diabetes. *Diabetes Care* 26:3215–3218.

Lee, P., and R. Chen. 2008. Vitamin D as an analgesic for patients with type 2 diabetes and neuropathic pain. *Archives of Internal Medicine* 168:771–772.

Lee, D. H., A. R. Folsom, L. Harnack et al. 2004. Does supplemental vitamin C increase cardiovascular disease risk in women with diabetes? *American Journal of Clinical Nutrition* 80:1194–1200.

Liu, R. 2003. Health benefits of fruit and vegetables are from additive and synergistic combinations of phytochemicals. *American Journal of Clinical Nutrition* 78:517S–520S.

Rabinovitz, H., A. Friedensohn, A. Leibovitz et al. 2004. Effect of chromium supplementation on blood glucose and lipid levels in type 2 diabetes mellitus elderly patients. *International Journal for Vitamin and Nutrition Research* 74:178–182.

Ruhe, R., R. McDonald. 2001. Use of antioxidant nutrients in the prevention and treatment of type 2 diabetes. *Journal of the American College of Nutrition* 20:363S–368S.

Schmid, U., H. Stopper, A. Heidland, N. Schupp. 2008. Benfotiamine exhibits direct antioxidative capacity and prevents induction of DNA damage in vitro. *Diabetes/Metabolism Research and Reviews,* April 2.

Sima, A. A., M. Calvani, M. Mehra et al. 2005. Acetyl-L-carnitine improves pain, nerve regeneration, and vibratory perception in patients with chronic diabetic neuropathy: An analysis of two randomized placebo-controlled trials. *Diabetes Care* 28:89–94.

Sugiura, M., M. Nakamura, Y. Ikoma et al. 2006. The homeostasis model assessment-insulin resistance index is inversely associated with serum carotenoids in non-diabetic subjects. *Journal of Epidemiology* 16:71–78.

Thornalley, P. J. 2005. The potential role of thiamine (vitamin B(1)) in diabetic complications. *Current Diabetes Reviews* 1:287–298.

Yeh, G., D. Eisenberg, T. Kaptchuk, R. Phillips. 2003. Systematic review of herbs and dietary supplements for glycemic control in diabetes. *Diabetes Care* 26:1277–1294.

Ziegler, D., A. Ametov, A. Barinov et al. 2006. Oral treatment with alpha-lipoic acid improves symptomatic diabetic polyneuropathy: The SYDNEY 2 trial. *Diabetes Care* 29:2365–2370.

Chapter 5: Moving More for Your Body, Heart, and Mind

American College of Sports Medicine. 2000. Exercise and type 2 diabetes. *Medicine & Science in Sports & Exercise* 32:1345–1360.

Borghouts, L., H. Keizer. 2000. Exercise and insulin sensitivity: A review. *International Journal of Sports Medicine* 21:1–12.

Brooks, N., J. E. Layne, P. L. Gordon et al. 2006. Strength training improves muscle quality and insulin sensitivity in Hispanic older adults with type 2 diabetes. *International Journal of Medical Sciences* 4:19–27.

Bruce, C., J. Hawley. 2004. Improvements in insulin resistance with aerobic exercise training: A lipocentric approach. *Medicine and Science in Sports and Exercise* 36:1196–1201.

Cuff, D. J., G. S. Meneilly, A. Martin et al. 2003. Effective exercise modality to reduce insulin resistance in women with type 2 diabetes. *Diabetes Care* 26:2977–2982.

Cukierman, T., H. C. Gerstein, J. D. Williamson. 2005. Cognitive decline and dementia in diabetes-systematic overview of prospective observational studies. *Diabetologia* 48:2460–2469.

Dela, F., K. J. Mikines, J. J. Larsen, H. Galbo. 1999. Glucose clearance in trained skeletal muscle during maximal insulin with superimposed exercise. *Journal of Applied Physiology* 87:2059–2067.

Dela, F., M. E. von Linstow, K. J. Mikines, H. Galbo. 2004. Physical training may enhance beta-cell function in type 2 diabetes. *American Journal of Physiology* 287:E1024–E1031.

Di Loreto, C., C. Fanelli, P. Lucidi et al. 2005. Make your diabetic patients walk: Long-term impact of different amounts of physical activity on type 2 diabetes. *Diabetes Care* 28:1295–1302.

Dunstan, D. W., R. M. Daly, N. Owen et al. 2002. High-intensity resistance training improves glycemic control in older patients with type 2 diabetes. *Diabetes Care* 25:1729–1736.

Dunstan, D. W., R. M. Daly, N. Owen et al. 2005. Home-based resistance training is not sufficient to maintain improved glycemic control following supervised training in older individuals with type 2 diabetes. *Diabetes Care* 28:3–9.

Ebeling, P., H. A. Koistinen, V. A. Koivisto. 1998. Insulin-independent glucose transport regulates insulin sensitivity. *FEBS Letters* 436:301–303.

Engel, L., H. Lindner. 2006. Impact of using a pedometer on time spent walking in older adults with type 2 diabetes. *Diabetes Educator* 32:98–107.

Fox, K. R. 1999. The influence of physical activity on mental well-being. *Public Health Nutrition* 2:411–418.

Giannopoulou, I., L. L. Ploutz-Synder, R. Carhart et al. 2005. Exercise is required for visceral fat loss in postmenopausal women with type 2 diabetes. *Journal of Clinical Endocrinology and Metabolism* 90:1511–1518.

Hamilton, M. T., D. G. Hamilton, T. W. Zderic. 2007. Role of low energy expenditure and sitting in obesity, metabolic syndrome, type 2 diabetes, and cardiovascular disease. *Diabetes* 56:2655–2667.

Haskell, W. L., I. M. Lee, R. R. Pate et al. 2007. Physical activity and public health: Updated recommendation for adults from the American College of Sports Medicine and the American Heart Association. *Medicine and Science in Sports and Exercise* 39:1423–1434.

Hawley, J. A. 2004. Exercise as a therapeutic intervention for the prevention and treatment of insulin resistance. *Diabetes/Metabolism Research and Reviews* 20:383–393.

Henriksen, E. J. 2006. Exercise training and the antioxidant alpha-lipoic acid in the treatment of insulin resistance and type 2 diabetes. *Free Radical Biology & Medicine* 40:3–12.

Houmard, J. A., C. J. Tanner, C. A. Slentz et al. 2004. Effect of the volume and intensity of exercise training on insulin sensitivity. *Journal of Applied Physiology* 96:101–106.

Hu, F. B., R. J. Sigal, J. W. Rich-Edwards et al. 1999. Walking compared with vigorous physical activity and risk of type 2 diabetes in women: A prospective study. *Journal of the American Medical Association* 282:1433–1439.

Hultquist, C. N., C. Albright, D. L. Thompson. 2005. Comparison of walking recommendations in previously inactive women. *Medicine and Science in Sports and Exercise* 37:676–683.

Ibañez, J., M. Izquierdo, I. Argüelles et al. 2005. Twice-weekly progressive resistance training decreases abdominal fat and improves insulin sensitivity in older men with type 2 diabetes. *Diabetes Care* 28:662–667.

Ishii, T., T. Yamakita, T. Sato et al. 1998. Resistance training improves insulin sensitivity in NIDDM subjects without altering maximal oxygen uptake. *Diabetes Care* 21:1351–1355.

Johnson, S. T., L. J. McCargar, G. J. Bell et al. 2006. Walking faster: Distilling a complex prescription for type 2 diabetes management through pedometry. *Diabetes Care* 29:1654–1655.

Kadoglou, N. P., F. Iliadis, N. Angelopoulou et al. 2007. The anti-inflammatory effects of exercise training in patients with type 2 diabetes mellitus. *European Journal of Cardiovascular Prevention and Rehabilitation* 14:637–643.

Knowler, W. C., E. Barrett-Connor, S. E. Fowler et al. 2002. Reduction in the incidence of type 2 diabetes with lifestyle intervention or metformin. *New England Journal of Medicine* 346:393–403.

Kubukeli, Z. N., T. D. Noakes, S. C. Dennis. 2002. Training techniques to improve endurance exercise performances. *Sports Medicine* 32:489–509.

Levine, J. A., S. J. Schleusner, M. D. Jensen. 2000. Energy expenditure of nonexercise activity. *American Journal of Clinical Nutrition* 72:1451–1454.

Mier, N., A. A. Medina, M. G. Ory. 2007. Mexican Americans with type 2 diabetes: Perspectives on definitions, motivators, and programs of physical activity. *Preventing Chronic Disease* 4:A24.

Nelson, M. E., W. J. Rejeski, S. N. Blair et al. 2007. Physical activity and public health in older adults: Recommendation from the American College of Sports Medicine and the American Heart Association. *Medicine and Science in Sports and Exercise* 39:1435–1445.

Penedo, F. J., J. R. Dahn. 2005. Exercise and well-being: A review of mental and physical health benefits associated with physical activity. *Current Opinion in Psychiatry* 18:189–193.

Petersen, A. M., B. K. Pedersen. 2005. The anti-inflammatory effect of exercise. *Journal of Applied Physiology* 98:1154–1162.

Poirier, P., S. Mawhinney, L. Gondin et al. 2001. Prior meal enhances the plasma glucose lowering effect of exercise in type 2 diabetes. *Medicine & Science in Sports & Exercise* 33:1259–1264.

Savage, D. B., K. F. Petersen, G. I. Shulman. 2005. Mechanisms of insulin resistance in humans and possible links with inflammation. *Hypertension* 45:828–833.

Sigal, R. J., G. P. Kenny, N. G. Boulé et al. 2007. Effects of aerobic training, resistance training, or both on glycemic control in type 2 diabetes: A randomized trial. *Annals of Internal Medicine* 147:357–369.

Sigal, R. J., G. P. Kenny, D. H. Wasserman et al. 2004. Physical activity/exercise and type 2 diabetes. *Diabetes Care* 27:2518–2538.

Sigal, R. J., G. P. Kenny, D. H. Wasserman et al. 2006. Physical activity/exercise and type 2 diabetes: A consensus statement from the American Diabetes Association. *Diabetes Care* 29:1433–1438.

Solomon, T. P., S. N. Sistrun, R. K. Krishnan et al. 2008. Exercise and diet enhance fat oxidation and reduce insulin resistance in older obese adults. *Journal of Applied Physiology* 104:1313–1319.

Su, F., Y. Y. Chang, H. H. Pai et al. 2004. Infusion of beta-endorphin improves insulin resistance in fructose-fed rats. *Hormone & Metabolism Research* 36:571–577.

Tuomilehto, J., J. Lindstrom, J. G. Eriksson et al. 2001. Prevention of type 2 diabetes mellitus by changes in lifestyle among subjects with impaired glucose tolerance. *New England Journal of Medicine* 344:1343–1350.

Voelker, R. 2006. Studies suggest dog walking a good strategy for fostering fitness. *Journal of the American Medical Association* 296:643.

Chapter 6: Learning How to Exercise Safely and Effectively

American College of Sports Medicine. 2000. Exercise and type 2 diabetes. *Medicine & Science in Sports & Exercise* 32:1345–1360.

Cryer, P. E. 2006. Hypoglycemia in diabetes: Pathophysiological mechanisms and diurnal variation. *Progress in Brain Research* 153:361–365.

Cukierman, T., H. C. Gerstein, J. D. Williamson. 2005. Cognitive decline and dementia in diabetes-systematic overview of prospective observational studies. *Diabetologia* 48:2460–2469.

Dela, F., K. J. Mikines, J. J. Larsen, H. Galbo. 1999. Glucose clearance in trained skeletal muscle during maximal insulin with superimposed exercise. *Journal of Applied Physiology* 87:2059–2067.

Dela, F., M. E. von Linstow, K. J. Mikines, H. Galbo. 2004. Physical training may enhance beta-cell function in type 2 diabetes. *American Journal of Physiology* 287:E1024–E1031.

Ebeling, P., H. A. Koistinen, V. A. Koivisto. 1998. Insulin-independent glucose transport regulates insulin sensitivity. *FEBS Letters* 436:301–303.

Haskell, W. L., I. M. Lee, R. R. Pate et al. 2007. Physical activity and public health: Updated recommendation for adults from the American College of Sports Medicine and the American Heart Association. *Medicine and Science in Sports and Exercise* 39:1423–1434.

Henderson, J. N., K. V. Allen, I. J. Deary, B. M. Frier. 2003. Hypoglycaemia in insulin-treated Type 2 diabetes: Frequency, symptoms, and impaired awareness. *Diabetic Medicine* 20:1016–1021.

Kadoglou, N. P., F. Iliadis, N. Angelopoulou et al. 2007. The anti-inflammatory effects of exercise training in patients with type 2 diabetes mellitus. *European Journal of Cardiovascular Prevention and Rehabilitation* 14:637–643.

Kubukeli, Z. N., T. D. Noakes, S. C. Dennis. 2002. Training techniques to improve endurance exercise performances. *Sports Medicine* 32:489–509.

Nelson, M. E., W. J. Rejeski, S. N. Blair et al. 2007. Physical activity and public health in older adults: Recommendation from the American College of Sports Medicine and the American Heart Association. *Medicine and Science in Sports and Exercise* 39:1435–1445.

Petersen, A. M., B. K. Pedersen. 2005. The anti-inflammatory effect of exercise. *Journal of Applied Physiology* 98:1154–1162.

Poirier, P., S. Mawhinney, L. Gondin et al. 2001. Prior meal enhances the plasma glucose lowering effect of exercise in type 2 diabetes. *Medicine & Science in Sports & Exercise* 33:1259–1264.

Praet, S. F., R. A. Jonkers, G. Schep et al. 2008. Long-standing, insulin-treated type 2 diabetes patients with complications respond well to short-term resistance and interval exercise training. *European Journal of Endocrinology* 158:163–172.

Sigal, R. J., G. P. Kenny, D. H. Wasserman et al. 2004. Physical activity/exercise and type 2 diabetes. *Diabetes Care* 27:2518–2538.

Sigal, R. J., G. P. Kenny, D. H. Wasserman et al. 2006. Physical activity/exercise and type 2 diabetes: A consensus statement from the American Diabetes Association. *Diabetes Care* 29:1433–1438.

Verghese, J. 2006. Cognitive and mobility profile of older social dancers. *Journal of the American Geriatric Society* 54:1241–1244.

Vincent, K. R., R. W. Braith, R. A. Feldman et al. 2002. Resistance exercise and physical performance in adults aged 60 to 83. *Journal of the American Geriatrics Society* 50:1100–1107.

Zainuddin, Z., M. Newton, P. Sacco, K. Nosaka. 2005. Effects of massage on delayed-onset muscle soreness, swelling, and recovery of muscle function. *Journal of Athletic Training* 40:174–180.

Chapter 7: Treating Your Diabetes Right: Monitoring and Medications

Bond, A. 2006. Exenatide (Byetta) as a novel treatment option for type 2 diabetes mellitus. *Proceedings* (Baylor University Medical Center) 19:281–284.

Buse, J. B., R. R. Henry, J. Han et al. 2004. Effects of exenatide (exendin-4) on glycemic control over 30 weeks in sulfonylurea-treated patients with type 2 diabetes. *Diabetes Care* 27:2628–2635.

Caballero, A. E. 2008. Long-term benefits of insulin therapy and glycemic control in overweight and obese adults with type 2 diabetes. *Journal of Diabetes and Its Complications* April 15.

Cook, M. N., C. J. Girman, P. P. Stein et al. 2005. Glycemic control continues to deteriorate after sulfonylureas are added to metformin among patients with type 2 diabetes. *Diabetes Care* 28:995–1000.

Dailey, G., J. Rosenstock, R. G. Moses et al. 2004. Insulin glulisine [Apidra] provides improved glycemic control in patients with type 2 diabetes. *Diabetes Care* 27:2363–2368.

Davidson, J. 2005. Strategies for improving glycemic control: Effective use of glucose monitoring. *American Journal of Medicine* 118:27S–32S.

Davis, S. N., S. M. Renda. 2006. Psychological insulin resistance: Overcoming barriers to starting insulin therapy. *Diabetes Educator* 32:146S–152S.

Garg, S. K., S. L. Ellis, H. Ulrich. 2005. Insulin glulisine: A new rapid-acting insulin analogue for the treatment of diabetes. *Expert Opinions in Pharmacotherapy* 6:643–651.

Green, B. D., P. R. Flatt, C. J. Bailey. 2006. Dipeptidyl peptidase IV (DPP IV) inhibitors: A newly emerging drug class for the treatment of type 2 diabetes. *Diabetes & Vascular Disease Research* 3:159–165.

Hallsten, K., K. A. Virtanen, F. Lonnqvist et al. 2002. Rosiglitazone but not metformin enhances insulin- and exercise-stimulated skeletal muscle glucose uptake in patients with newly diagnosed type 2 diabetes. *Diabetes* 51:3479–3485.

Herman, W. H., L. L. Ilag, S. L. Johnson et al. 2005. A clinical trial of continuous subcutaneous insulin infusion versus multiple daily injections in older adults with type 2 diabetes. *Diabetes Care* 28:1568–1573.

Joy, S. V., P. T. Rodgers, A. C. Scates. 2005. Incretin mimetics as emerging treatment for type 2 diabetes. *Annals of Pharmacotherapy* 39:110–118.

Kendall, D. M., M. C. Riddle, J. Rosenstock et al. 2005. Effects of exenatide (exendin-4) on glycemic control over 30 weeks in patients with type 2 diabetes treated with metformin and a sulfonylurea. *Diabetes Care* 28:1083–1091.

Kirk, J. K., L. V. Passmore, R. A. Bell et al. 2008. Disparities in A1C levels between Hispanic and non-Hispanic white adults with diabetes: A meta-analysis. *Diabetes Care* 31:240–246.

Larsen, J., F. Dela, S. Madsbad et al. 1999. Interaction of sulfonylureas and exercise on glucose homeostasis in type 2 diabetic patients. *Diabetes Care* 22:1647–1654.

Martin, S., B. Schneider, L. Heinemann et al. 2006. Self-monitoring of blood glucose in type 2 diabetes and long-term outcome: An epidemiological cohort study. *Diabetologia* 49:271–278.

Moon, R. J., L. A. Bascombe, R. I. Holt. 2007. The addition of metformin in type 1 diabetes improves insulin sensitivity, diabetic control, body composition, and patient well-being. *Diabetes, Obesity & Metabolism* 9:143–145.

Murata, G. H., J. H. Shah, R. M. Hoffman et al. 2003. Intensified blood glucose monitoring improves glycemic control in stable, insulin-treated veterans with type 2 diabetes: The Diabetes Outcomes in Veterans Study (DOVES). *Diabetes Care* 26:1759–1763.

Nathan, D. M., J. Kuenen, R. Borg et al. 2008. Translating the A1C assay into estimated average glucose values. *Diabetes Care* 31:1473–1478.

Peterson, G. E. 2006. Intermediate and long-acting insulins: A review of NPH insulin, insulin glargine and insulin detemir. *Current Medical Research and Opinion* 22:2613–2619.

Raskin, P., E. Allen, P. Hollander et al. 2005. Initiating insulin therapy in type 2 diabetes: A comparison of biphasic and basal insulin analogs. *Diabetes Care* 28:260–265.

Reusch, J. E., J. G. Regensteiner, P. A. Watson. 2003. Novel actions of thiazolidinediones on vascular function and exercise capacity. *American Journal of Medicine* 115:69S–74S.

Ryan, E., S. Imes, C. Wallace. 2001. Short-term intensity insulin therapy in newly diagnosed type 2 diabetes. *Diabetes Care* 27:1028–1032.

Sarol, J. N., N. A. Nicodemus, K. M. Tan, M. B. Grava. 2005. Self-monitoring of blood glucose as part of a multi-component therapy among non-insulin requiring type 2 diabetes patients: A meta-analysis (1966–2004). *Current Medical Research and Opinion* 21:173–184.

Chapter 8: Controlling Stress, Depression, and Your Emotions

Avena, N. M., P. Rada, B. G. Hoebel. 2008. Evidence for sugar addiction: Behavioral and neurochemical effects of intermittent, excessive sugar intake. *Neuroscience and Biobehavioral Reviews* 32:20-39.

Ciechanowski, P. S., W. J. Katon, J. E. Russo. 2000. Depression and diabetes: Impact of depressive symptoms on adherence, function, and costs. *Archives of Internal Medicine* 160:3278–3285.

Clark, A., A. Seidler, M. Miller. 2001. Inverse association between sense of humor and coronary heart disease. *International Journal of Cardiology* 80:87–88.

Egede, L. E. 2005. Effect of comorbid chronic diseases on prevalence and odds of depression in adults with diabetes. *Psychometric Medicine* 67:46–51.

Hayashi, K., T. Hayashi, S. Iwanaga et al. 2003. Laughter lowered the increase in postprandial blood glucose. *Diabetes Care* 26:1651–1652.

Krein, S. L., M. Heisler, J. D. Piette et al. 2005. The effect of chronic pain on diabetes patients' self-management. *Diabetes Care* 28:65–70.

Nasir, U. M., S. Iwanaga, A. H. Nabi et al. 2005. Laughter therapy modulates the parameters of renin-angiotensin system in patients with type 2 diabetes. *International Journal of Molecular Medicine* 16:1077–1081.

Park, H., Y. Hong, H. Lee, E. Ha, Y. Sung. 2004. Individuals with type 2 diabetes and depressive symptoms exhibited lower adherence with self-care. *Journal of Clinical Epidemiology* 57:978–984.

Peyrot, M., J. F. McMurry Jr., D. F. Kruger. 1999. A biopsychosocial model of glycemic control in diabetes: Stress, coping and regimen adherence. *Journal of Health and Social Behavior* 40:141–158.

Pibernik-Okanovic, M., M. Prasek et al. 2004. Effects of an empowerment-based psychosocial intervention on quality of life and metabolic control in type 2 diabetic patients. *Patient Education and Counseling* 52:193–199.

Raji, M. A., C. A. Reyes-Ortiz, Y. F. Kuo et al. 2007. Depressive symptoms and cognitive change in older Mexican Americans. *Journal of Geriatric Psychiatry and Neurology* 20:145–152.

Reyes-Ortiz, C. A., I. M. Berges, M. A. Raji et al. 2008. Church attendance mediates the association between depressive symptoms and cognitive functioning among older Mexican Americans. *Journals of Gerontology*. Series A, Biological Sciences and Medical Sciences 63:480–486.

Rose, M., H. Fliege, M. Hildebrandt et al. 2002. The network of psychological variables in patients with diabetes and their importance for quality of life and metabolic control. *Diabetes Care* 25:35–42.

Rotkiewicz-Piorun, A. M., S. Al Snih, M. A. Raji et al. 2006. Cognitive decline in older Mexican Americans with diabetes. *Journal of the National Medical Association* 98:1840–1847.

Surwit, R. S., M. A. van Tilburg, N. Zucker et al. 2002. Stress management improves long-term glycemic control in type 2 diabetes. *Diabetes Care* 25:30–34.

Taylor-Piliae, R. E., W. L. Haskell, C. M. Waters, E. S. Froelicher. 2006. Change in perceived psychosocial status following a 12-week Tai Chi exercise program. *Journal of Advanced Nursing* 54:313–329.

Timonen, M., M. Laakso, J. Jokelainen et al. 2005. Insulin resistance and depression: Cross sectional study. *British Medical Journal* 330:17–18.

Trief, P. M., R. Ploutz-Snyder, K. D. Britton, R. S. Weinstock. 2004. The relationship between marital quality and adherence to the diabetes care regimen. *Annals of Behavioral Medicine* 27:148–154.

Turan, B., Z. Osar, J. Molzan Turan et al. 2002. The role of coping with disease in adherence to treatment regimen and disease control in type 1 and insulin treated type 2 diabetes mellitus. *Diabetes & Metabolism* 28:186–193.

Van Dam, H. A., F. G. van der Horst, L. Knoops et al. 2005. Social support in diabetes: A systematic review of controlled intervention studies. *Patient Education and Counseling* 59:1–12.

Zhang, X., S. L. Norris, E. W. Gregg et al. 2005. Depressive symptoms and mortality among persons with and without diabetes. *American Journal of Epidemiology* 161:652–660.

Chapter 9: Limiting Diabetes-Related Health Problems

American Diabetes Association. When You Travel. http://www.diabetes.org/pre-diabetes/travel/when-you-travel.jsp.

Balducci, S., G. Iacobellis, L. Parisi et al. 2006. Exercise training can modify the natural history of diabetic peripheral neuropathy. *Journal of Diabetes and Its Complications* 20:216–223.

Briggs, J. E., P. P. McKeown, V. L. Crawford et al. 2006. Angiographically confirmed coronary heart disease and periodontal disease in middle-aged males. *Journal of Periodontology* 77:95–102.

Ceriello, A. 2003. The possible role of postprandial hyperglycaemia in the pathogenesis of diabetic complications. *Diabetologia* 46:M9–M16.

Dairman, T. 2006. Diabetes resources: Travel tips. *Diabetes Self-Management* 23:64–65.

Dobretsov, M., D. Romanovsky, J. R. Stimers. 2007. Early diabetic neuropathy: Triggers and mechanisms. *World Journal of Gastroenterology* 13:175–191.

Hirsch, I. B. 2005. Intensifying insulin therapy in patients with type 2 diabetes mellitus. *American Journal of Medicine* 118:21S–26S.

Kirk, J. K., L. V. Passmore, R. A. Bell et al. 2008. Disparities in A1C levels between Hispanic and non-Hispanic white adults with diabetes: A meta-analysis. *Diabetes Care* 31:240–246.

Lee, P., R. Chen. 2008. Vitamin D as an analgesic for patients with type 2 diabetes and neuropathic pain. *Archives of Internal Medicine* 168:771–772.

Lumber, T., P. A. Strainic. 2005. Have insulin, will travel: Planning ahead will make traveling with insulin smooth sailing. *Diabetes Forecast* 58:50–54.

Manley, S. 2003. Haemoglobin A1c—A marker for complications of type 2 diabetes: The experience from the UK Prospective Diabetes Study (UKPDS). *Clinical Chemistry and Laboratory Medicine* 41:1182–1190.

Mealey, B. L., T. W. Oates et al. 2006. Diabetes mellitus and periodontal diseases. *Journal of Periodontology* 77:1289–1303.

Pop-Busui, R., A. Sima, M. Stevens. 2006. Diabetic neuropathy and oxidative stress. *Diabetes/Metabolism Research and Reviews* 22:257–273.

Praet, S. F., R. A. Jonkers, G. Schep et al. 2008. Long-standing, insulin-treated type 2 diabetes patients with complications respond well to short-term resistance and interval exercise training. *European Journal of Endocrinology* 158:163–172.

Whiteley, L., S. Padmanabhan, D. Hole et al. 2005. Should diabetes be considered a coronary heart disease risk equivalent? *Diabetes Care* 28:1588–1593.

Yun, K. E., M. J. Park, H. S. Park. 2007. Lack of management of cardiovascular risk Factors in type 2 diabetic patients. *International Journal of Clinical Practice* 61:39–44.

Chapter 10: Staying on the Road to Good Health

Begley S. 2007. How the brain rewires itself. *Time*, January 29.

De Cosmo, S., O. Lamacchia, A. Rauseo et al. 2006. Cigarette smoking is associated with low glomerular filtration rate in male patients with type 2 diabetes. *Diabetes Care* 29:2467–2470.

Deshpande, A. D., E. A. Baker, S. L. Lovegreen, R. C. Brownson. 2005. Environmental correlates of physical activity among individuals with diabetes in the rural Midwest. *Diabetes Care* 28:1012–1018.

Di Loreto, C., C. Fanelli, P. Lucidi et al. 2005. Make your diabetic patients walk: Long-term impact of different amounts of physical activity on type 2 diabetes. *Diabetes Care* 28:1295–1302.

Eliasson, B. 2003. Cigarette smoking and diabetes. *Progress in Cardiovascular Diseases* 45:405–413.

Estabrooks, P. A., C. C. Nelson, S. Xu et al. 2005. The frequency and behavioral outcomes of goal choices in the self-management of diabetes. *Diabetes Educator* 31:391–400.

Grossman, M. D., A. L. Stewart. 2003. "You aren't going to get better by just sitting around": Physical activity perceptions, motivations, and barriers in adults 75 years of age or older. *American Journal of Geriatric Cardiology* 12:33–37.

Hyman, J. J., D. M. Winn, B. C. Reid. 2002. The role of cigarette smoking in the association between periodontal disease and coronary heart disease. *Journal of Periodontology* 73:988–994.

Ilies, R., T. A. Judge. 2005. Goal regulation across time: The effects of feedback and affect. *Journal of Applied Psychology* 90:453–467.

Lerman, I., L. Lozano, A. R. Villa et al. 2004. Psychosocial factors associated with poor diabetes self-care management in a specialized center in Mexico City. *Biomedicine and Pharmacotherapy* 58:566–570.

Rose, M., H. Fliege, M. Hildebrandt et al. 2002. The network of psychological variables in patients with diabetes and their importance for quality of life and metabolic control. *Diabetes Care* 25:35–42.

Seefeldt, V., R. M. Malina, and M. A. Clark. 2002. Factors affecting levels of physical activity in adults. *Sports Medicine* 32:143–168.

Skinner, T. C. 2004. Psychological barriers. *European Journal of Endocrinology* 151:T13–T17.

Sprague, M. A., J. A. Shultz, L. J. Branen. 2006. Understanding patient experiences with goal setting for diabetes self-management after diabetes education. *Family & Community Health* 29:245–255.

Van Dam, H. A., F. G. van der Horst, L. Knoops et al. 2005. Social support in diabetes: A systematic review of controlled intervention studies. *Patient Education and Counseling* 59:1–12.

Yates, L. B., L. Djoussé, T. Kurth et al. 2008. Exceptional longevity in men: Modifiable factors associated with survival and function to age 90 years. *Archives of Internal Medicine* 168:284–290.

Conclusion: Taking on Diabetes . . . and Winning

Colberg, S. R., S. V. Edelman. *50 Secrets of the Longest Living People with Diabetes.* New York: Marlowe, 2007.

Yates, L. B., L. Djoussé, T. Kurth et al. 2008. Exceptional longevity in men: Modifiable factors associated with survival and function to age 90 years. *Archives of Internal Medicine* 168:284–290.

ACKNOWLEDGMENTS

Creating a quality book is a group project, and we have *muchas personas* to thank for helping us. First and foremost, our thanks go to the diabetic Latinos and Latinas who were willing to share their stories with us (thereby breaking the usual Latino rule of denying their diabetes and not sharing it with anyone). Acting as role models for the rest of the Latino community, these individuals are inspirational in their own right as champions for the cause. We also thank Marina Moure, who reviewed this book for us with fresh Latina eyes.

Along a similar vein, we owe a debt of gratitude to celebrity Latina Chef LaLa for her service in taking on diabetes for the Latino community with delicious and healthy cooking even though she is diabetes-free herself and for taking the time to write such an inspiring foreword for this book. Thank you, LaLa. We feel fortunate to be counted among your *amigos*.

We also owe a great deal to the hard-working crew members at Da Capo Press who kept this book moving forward. They include publisher and editor extraordinaire Matthew Lore, Wendy Francis, Wendie Carr, Julia Hall, Collin Tracy, and many, many others.

Last but not least, our agent, Linda Konner, found the best possible publisher for this book. We thank her for her efforts and for supporting this book idea from the start. Thanks, Linda. We could not have succeeded without your support and your expertise.

ABOUT THE AUTHORS

Sheri R. Colberg, PhD, is an exercise physiologist and professor of exercise science at Old Dominion University in Norfolk, Virginia, as well as an adjunct professor of internal medicine at Eastern Virginia Medical School. A respected researcher and lecturer, she has authored more than 150 research and educational articles on exercise, diabetes, and health, as well as numerous books, including *Diabetes-Free Kids, The 7 Step Diabetes Fitness Plan, 50 Secrets of the Longest Living People with Diabetes, The Science of Staying Young,* and *Diabetic Athlete's Handbook.* Her informative articles are available on her website at www.shericolberg.com. As executive director of the Lifelong Exercise Institute (www.lifelongexercise.com) and director of exercise physiology for Insulite Laboratories (www.insulite labs.com), she shares her knowledge about physical activity and healthy lifestyle habits with countless others. She also has more than forty years of personal experience as a type 1 diabetic exerciser who enjoys conditioning machines, swimming, biking, walking, tennis, weight training, hiking, and yard work, as well as playing soccer with her husband and three sons.

Leonel Villa-Caballero, MD, PhD, was born in Mexico City. A researcher and clinician in the Family and Preventive Medicine Department at the University of California–San Diego School of Medicine, he has more than fifteen years of experience treating patients with diabetes. Currently he serves as director of the Latino Initiative of Taking Control of your Diabetes (TCOYD), a notprofit organization that educates and empowers people with diabetes. As a result of his commitment to improving the health of the Latino community, he received the American Diabetes

Association's Cielo Award in 2006 and was recognized in America's Top Physicians in 2007. With his expertise in cultural aspects of Latino health, he is an investigator for various federal research grant projects and serves as a consultant to various biomedical companies focused on Latino health care issues. He currently resides in San Diego, California.

INDEX

A1c. *See* HbA1c
ACE-inhibitors, 168, 197
Acetyl-L-carnitine, 96–97, 98
Acidity and GI value, 54
Activity-related injuries, 111
Actos, 154, 155, 157, 162
Addiction to sugar, 61
Adhesive capsulitis (frozen shoulder), 97,
    117, 143–144
Adipocytes, 24
Adiponectin, 24
Adipose tissue, 7–8, 35–36. *See also* Body
    fat
Adrenaline, 103
Aerobic activities, 110–112, 134–135, 137,
    197–198, 214–215
Aging
    and alpha lipoic acid, 82–83
    and antioxidants, 45, 73
    changes from diabetes versus, 217–218
    Latino view of, 69–70
    losing muscle mass, 114–115, 217
    physical activity for slowing, 211–212
    stress leading to, 174–175
Albumin levels in urine, 142–143, 197
Alcohol, 125
All-you-can-eat buffets, 65–66
Alpha linolenic acid (ALA), 50
Alpha lipoic acid (LA), 73–74, 82–83, 98
Alpha-glucosidase inhibitors, 155, 158,
    162

Alzheimer's disease, 183
Amaryl, 154, 155, 156, 161–162
American Association of Diabetes
    Educators, 17
American Diabetes Association, 6, 42, 138,
    203, 204
American Heart Association, 50
Amino acids, 95–96
Amputations, 15, 138, 192, 195
Amylin, 155, 160, 162–163
Angina during exercise, 134–135
Anthocyanin, 44
Anticoagulants, 199
Anti-inflammatory diet, 41–42
Anti-inflammatory hormone, 56
Anti-inflammatory medications, 97, 144,
    145, 199. *See also* Aspirin therapy
Antioxidants
    benefits for diabetics, 73–74
    for dementia prevention, 183
    glutathione, 73–74, 82–83, 99
    glutatione peroxidase enzyme, 87
    overdosing dangers, 99
    overview, 44–45
    for peripheral neuropathy pain, 98, 99
    pycnogenol, 91
    quercetin, 97
    supplements, 73–74
    vitamin C, 73–74, 77, 79
    vitamin E, 73–74, 76, 81–82
Antiplatelet agents, 199

Apidra, 164–165
ARBS (angiotensin receptor blockers),
    197
Arthritis, 143–144
Artificial or low-calorie sweeteners, 62
Ascorbic acid (vitamin C), 73–74, 77, 79
Aspartame (NutraSweet), 62
Aspirin therapy
    and cinnamon, 91
    with Coumadin, warning about, 82
    for diabetes, 198
    and exercise, 144, 169
    and gamma-linolenic acid, 92
    for stroke prevention, 199
Autonomic nerve damage, 139–140, 195.
    See also Peripheral neuropathy
Avandia, 154, 155, 157, 162

B vitamins, 75, 78, 98
Babies of diabetic mothers, 201–202
Barbiturates and heliotropium, 70
Basal insulin, 164
Basal-bolus regimens, 164, 166, 167
Benfotiamine, 78, 98
Berberine from Rhizoma coptidis, 93–94
Beta cells, 2, 3, 90, 165, 179
Beta-blockers, 168
Beta-carotene, 73–74
Beyond Beans and Rice (Drago), 59
Biguanides, 11, 153–154, 155, 156–157
Binge-eating disorders, 183–184
Bioactive phenols in cinnamon, 90–91
Bioflavonoids, 91
Biotin, 75, 77, 78
Bitter melon (Momordica charantia),
    93–94
Blindness, 15, 79, 194, 198
Blood creatinine levels, 197
Blood glucose
    and GI tables, 54
    and magnesium, 86
    and periodontal disease, 199, 201
    stored in muscles, 7–8, 34–35, 58,
        103–104, 217
    strategies for controlling, 63
    uptake rate, 26

Blood glucose levels
    and caffeine, 64
    and exercise, 102–105
    hyperglycemia, 2, 72, 78, 104, 164
    importance of controlling, xv–xvi, 188,
        191–195
    insulin for lowering at rest, 104
    overview, 147
    and specific foods, 42
    during surgery, 10
    target goals, 154
    and timing of exercise, 120
    See also HbA1c; Hyperglycemia;
        Hypoglycemia; Monitoring your blood
        sugar; Spikes in blood glucose
Blood pressure
    diabetes management for controlling,
        132
    effects of exercise, 135, 137, 139,
        141–142, 168
    and ginseng, 70
    and laughter, 173
    and life span, 196–197
    low blood pressure, 168
    and medications, 168–169
    and peripheral artery disease, 137
    target goals, 154
    See also High blood pressure
Blood sugar level checks, 11. *See also*
    Monitoring your blood sugar
Blood tests
    A1c, 6
    for determining type of diabetes, 4
    fasting blood glucose, 4, 6
    oral glucose tolerance test, 6, 7
Blood thinners, 82, 91, 92, 169
Blue-purple foods, 44
Body fat
    as early symptom of disease, 117
    fitness as priority over losing, 28, 29,
        101, 118
    and insulin, 7–8
    relationship to diabetes, 21–22, 36
    storage of, 24–26, 34–36
    utilizing during recovery from exercise,
        104

visceral, 21–22, 24–26, 118
See also Weight loss
Body fat patterning, 25
Bolus doses, 166–167
Books on diabetes, 231–232
Borage oil, 98
Breakfast, 66
Byetta, 155, 160–161

Calcitriol (vitamin D), 76, 80–81, 98
Calcium, 80, 88
Calories, portion size, and carbohydrates
    list, 57–58
Cancer, selenium for preventing, 87
Capsaicin, 43–44, 92–93, 98
Carbohydrates
    dietary recommendations, 40–41
    and gastroparesis, 139, 197
    and glycemic index, 47–48, 52–55,
        52–56, 58, 228–229
    glycemic load of, 55–56, 185, 228–229
    for hypoglycemia treatment, 126
    and insulin, 26, 56, 104–105
    L-carnitine for metabolizing, 96–97
    portion size, calories, and, 57–58
    as primary fuel during exercise,
        103–104
    spikes from, 35–36, 41, 56, 183
Cardiac rehabilitation exercise programs,
    134
Cardiovascular diseases (CVD), 193–194,
    198–199. *See also* Heart diseases
Carnitine, 96–97
Carotenoids, 44, 74–75
Carpal tunnel syndrome, 117
Cataracts, 79, 83, 140
Causes of diabetes, 15, 22
Center for Food Safety and Applied
    Nutrition (FDA), 94
Certified diabetes educators (CDEs), 17,
    59–60, 131–133
Chair exercises, 112–113
Cherries, tart, 44
Children of diabetic individuals, 201–202
China study, 31
Chocolate, 45, 126, 182

Cholesterol
    eliminating saturated and trans fat, 52
    and fiber, 47
    HDL, 27
    LDL, 48–49, 51, 90
    and liver, 27
    purpose and sources of, 52
    and sedentary lifestyle, 34
    statins for treating, 153, 167–168
    target goals, 154
Chromium, 83, 85–86, 88
Chromium picolinate, 78, 86
Cienfuegos, Socorro, 187–188
Cinnamon, 90–91
Clinical Center for National Institutes of
    Health, 94
Coffee, 45, 64
Color of foods, 44, 49, 74–75
Combination medication therapies, 154,
    156, 158–160, 164–165
Community, fun activities in the, 210,
    213–214
Complications. *See* Diabetes
    complications
Cooking methods, x–xi, 45–46, 54
Copper, 73–74, 89
Cortez, José, 31–32
Cortisol, 103, 174–175, 179
Coumadin, 82, 92, 169, 199
Coumarins in cinnamon, 91
C-peptide levels, 177
C-reactive protein, 95
Creatine supplements, 95–96
Crestor, 153, 167–168
Cross training, 145–146
Cuban Americans, xv. *See also* Latinos
Cultural heritage
    chubby babies are healthier than thin
        babies, 21, 27
    denial as part of, 10–11, 187
    and eliminating sugar, 9, 11
    fear of insulin, 163
    good eating and little exercise, 101
    herbal and folk medicines, 69–70
    myths and beliefs, 15–16
    See also Family; Latinos

CVD (cardiovascular diseases), 193–194, 198–199. *See also* Heart diseases
Cymbalta, 197

Daily tasks and chores
breaking large goals into, 211, 215–216
checking your feet, 138, 141
journals, 217
mental activity, 181–182
oral hygiene, 199, 201
overview, 8
small changes in daily habits, 29–30, 119, 208–209
See also Diabetes management; Exercise; Healthy eating; Monitoring your blood sugar
Dairy products, 48, 49, 51, 96–97, 127
Dancing as aerobic exercise, 111, 112, 214–215
Deaths from diabetes, xvi, 172, 191–196, 217–218
Dehydration prevention, 129–130
Delayed-onset muscle soreness (DOMS), 144–145
Dementia, 183
Denial in Latino culture, 10–11, 187
Depression, 175–176. *See also* Stress
Dermatitis from mugwort, 70
DHA (docosahexaenoic acid), 49, 50
DiaBeta, 154, 155, 156, 161–162
Diabetes, consequences of not controlling, xv–xvi. *See also* Diabetes complications; Diabetes management
Diabetes, potential cure with capsaicin, 93
Diabetes, statistics on incidence of, ix, xiv–xv, 195–196. *See also* Type 1 diabetes; Type 2 diabetes
Diabetes Care, 118
Diabetes complications
amputations, 15, 138, 192, 195
blindness, 15, 79, 194, 198
foot ulcers, 98–99, 138–139, 195
kidney disease, 142–143, 194–195
Latinos' likelihood of dying from, 195–196
nerve damage, 139–140, 195

nonprescription treatments for, 97–100
overview, xvi, 191–195
precautions for exercising with, 141
risk of dying from, 193–194
See also Heart diseases
Diabetes diagnosis, 5–8
Diabetes education classes, 16, 60
Diabetes educators, 17, 59–60, 131–133
Diabetes Hands Foundation, 178
Diabetes management
discipline and mental control for, 159
empowering yourself with knowledge, 208
Gloria Rodriguez's story, 9–12
overcoming barriers to exercise, 208–214
overview, 204–205, 221–222
rewarding yourself for your success, 215–216
self-care on bad days, 216–217
smoking cessation, 137, 181, 218–219
strategies for controlling blood sugar, 63
suggestions from successful diabetics, 11, 32, 84–85, 107–108, 132–133, 159, 178–179, 200
taking daily steps, 208–209
See also Daily tasks and chores; Doctors; Exercise; Medications; Monitoring your blood sugar
Diabetes prevention in the Latino community, 31–32
Diabetes Prevention Program, 30–31, 118
Diabetes Prevention Program (DPP), xv
Diabetic Athlete's Handbook (Colberg), 125
Diabetic ulcers, 98–99, 138–139, 195
Diabinese, 154, 155, 156, 161–162
Diagnosing diabetes, 4–8
Dialysis and exercise, 142
Dietary styles
anti-inflammatory, 41–42
beyond beans and rice, 59–60
fast food, 34, 41, 48–49
grazing, 66
inflammatory, 41, 48, 50
low-fat, 31, 39, 51, 63
sugar-free foods, 61–62
See also Healthy eating; Processed foods

Dieting, x, 27–28, 183–184
Discipline, 159
Diseases, 23–24, 47. *See also* Diabetes
  complications; High blood pressure
Diuretics, 168
Doctors
  English as barrier to seeing, 13–14
  and exercise program, 121–122, 162
  finding a good fit for you, 16–17, 108,
    187, 208, 218
  importance of, 16–19, 215, 218
  informing about herbals and
    supplements, 70–71, 78, 82, 92–93,
    100
  in Mexico, 85
  ophthalmologists, 142, 198
  for pain or injuries during exercise,
    135–136, 145
  regular visits to, 200
  seeing (or not) before exercise, 121–122
  See also Medications
DOMS (delayed-onset muscle soreness),
  144–145
Dopamine, 183
DPP-4 inhibitors, 155, 157–158
Drago, Lorena, 59–60
DVDs for workouts, 112–113
Dvorak, Carmen, 131–133

EAG (estimated average glucose),
  151–152
Eating disorders, 183–184
Eating well. *See* Healthy eating
Eggs, 52
Electrolytes, 131
Emotions, 159, 172–173, 174–175,
  179–180
Endorphins, 180
Energy from physical activity, 210
English language barrier, 13–14
Environmental factors and diabetes,
  22–23, 30–31. *See also* Lifestyle
  choices
EPA (eicosapentaenoic acid), 49, 50
Epinephrine, 103
Erectile dysfunction, 91, 195

Estimated average glucose (eAG),
  151–152
EsTuDiabetes.com community, 178
Ethnic group classifications, xiii–xiv
Exercise
  as activities throughout the day, 106,
    108–110
  and antioxidant enzymes systems, 73
  benefits from, 97, 101–102, 179–180
  and blood glucose levels, 102–105
  fitness as priority over weight loss,
    23–24, 28, 29, 101, 118
  and HDL cholesterol, 49
  and insulin, 7–8, 104–106, 113–115
  intensity of, 105–106, 168, 210, 216–217
  and medications, 125, 161–162, 167–168
  overcoming barriers to, 208–214
  overview, 120
  rewarding yourself for success, 215–216
  statistics on Americans, 33
  time of day for, 120
  and weight loss, 24, 30–31, 117–119
  See also Exercising safely; Muscles
Exercise, types of
  aerobic, 110–112, 134–135, 137,
    197–198, 214–215
  cross training, 145–146
  interval training, 115–116
  resistance training, 95–96, 212
  stretching, 110, 116–117, 143–144
  swimming or pool exercises, 111–112
  weight training, 103, 113–115, 135,
    141–142
  See also Walking
Exercising safely
  doctor visit prior to starting, 121–122
  with eye disease, 140–142
  fluid intake, 129–131
  with heart disease, 134–136
  with high blood pressure, 137
  and high blood sugar, 129
  hypoglycemia and its symptoms,
    123–125
  hypoglycemia unawareness warning,
    127–128
  with kidney disease, 142–143

Exercising safely (*continued*)
    with leg pain, 136–137
    and muscle soreness, 144–146
    with nerve damage, 139–140
    overview, 121, 134, 146–147
    with peripheral neuropathy, 138–139
    tips for, 146
    treatments for hypoglycemia, 125–127
Eye diseases
    blindness from, 15, 79, 194, 198
    exercising safely with, 140–142
    from glutathione deficiency, 73–74, 83, 99
    and omega-3 essential fats, 50
    ophthalmologists and medical treatment, 142, 198
    overview, xvi
    preventing, 79, 87, 91
    proliferative diabetic retinopathy, xvi, 75, 140–142, 194, 198

Family
    and fun activities in your community, 213–214
    importance in Hispanic culture, xi, 12–13
    pregnancy with diabetes, 85, 158, 201–202
    support from, 102, 186–189, 200, 210, 212
    See also Cultural heritage
Farm-raised fish, 50
Fast food restaurants, 34, 41, 48–49
Fasting blood glucose level, 4, 6, 7
Fat-free foods, 61–62
Fats in foods, 48–52, 96–97, 126, 127. *See also* Body fat
Fernandez Silva, Emma, 187–188
Fiber, 46–48, 65–66
Fibrinogen, 201
Finnish Diabetes Prevention Study, 31
Fish and fish oils, 49, 50
Fit4D.com, 17
Fitness as priority over weight loss, 23–24, 28, 29, 101, 118. *See also* Exercise; Exercising safely

Flavonoids. *See* Antioxidants
Fluid intake, 129–131
Folate, 75, 77, 78
Folk medicine, 69–70
Food. *See* Healthy eating
Food and Drug Administration (FDA), 70, 94
Food preparation, x–xi, 45–46, 54
Foods, color of, 44, 49, 74–75
Foot ulcers, 98–99, 138–139, 195
Free radicals, 73, 183
Frozen shoulder (adhesive capsulitis), 97, 117, 143–144
Fruit juice, 61
Fruits, 43–45, 53, 55, 183

Gamma-linolenic acid (GLA), 92
Garcia, Marilyn, 107–108
Gastroparesis, 139, 158, 160, 195, 197
Genetics
    and body fat patterning, 25
    and capacity to feel happy, 173
    effectiveness of lifestyle changes, 30–31
    influence on diabetes development, 22–23, 36
    predisposition to diabetes, 2–4, 32, 159
Gestational diabetes, 4
GI (glycemic index), 47, 52–56, 58, 228–229
Gingko biloba, 91–92
Ginseng, 70, 93–94
GLA (gamma-linolenic acid), 92
Glaucoma, 79
Glucagon, 102–104
Glucophage, 11, 153–154, 155, 156–157
Glucose, 53. *See also* Blood glucose
Glucose intolerance, 23
Glucose tablets, 126
Glucose-raising hormones from exercise, 102–104
Glucotrol, 154, 155, 156, 161–162
Glumetza, 155, 156–157
Glutathione, 73–74, 82–83, 99
Glutathione peroxidase enzyme, 87
Glycated hemoglobin test. *See* HbA1c
Glycation end products, 78

Glycemic effect, 43
Glycemic index (GI), 47, 52–56, 58,
    228–229
Glycemic load (GL), 55–56, 185, 228–229
Glynase, 154, 155, 156, 161–162
Glyset, 155, 158, 162
Goals, sticking with, 215–216
Golfing, 214
Gómez Hoyos, Mariana, 84–85
Grazing, 66
Green foods, 44, 49
Group stress management program,
    172–173
Growth hormone, 103
Gum disease, 199, 201
Gym workouts, 180–181, 212

HbA1c (glycated hemoglobin test; A1c for
    short)
    estimated average glucose interpretation,
        151–152
    goal for test results, 151, 154
    of Latinos, 14, 149, 196
    overview, 6
HDL cholesterol, 27
Health complication avoidance, 8–9,
    13–15. *See also* Diabetes complications;
    Exercise; Healthy eating; Medications
Health-related excuses for failure to
    exercise, xi, 134, 211–212. *See also*
    Exercising safely
Healthy eating
    amount of food, 185–186
    anti-inflammatory diet, 41–42
    balancing food groups, 40–43
    and color of foods, 44, 49, 74–75
    cooking methods, x–xi, 45–46, 54
    dietary sources of vitamins and minerals,
        76–77, 88–89
    diets versus, x–xi, 27–28
    eating disorders versus, 183–184
    fats, 48–52
    fiber, 46–48, 65–66
    finding nutrient content in foods, 94
    food choice challenges, 59
    fruits, 43–45, 53, 55, 183

    fruits and vegetables, 43–45, 53, 55, 183
    glycemic index and glycemic load, 47,
        52–58, 185, 228–229
    grazing, 66
    for keeping weight off, 29–30, 31
    by Latina living with type 1 diabetes for
        over 50 years, 107–108
    for mood adjustments, 182–183
    overview, 37, 65–66, 67
    portion control and carb counting, 214
    preparation for, 212
    and supplements, 71
    tips for preparing healthier meals, 45–46
    vegetables, 43–45, 53, 65, 83, 212
    See also Supplements
Heart attack warning signs, 136, 198–199
Heart diseases
    exercising safely with, 134–136
    from inflammatory process, 48–49
    and insulin-resistant liver, 27
    medical treatments for, 198–199
    and omega-3 essential fats, 50
    overview, 193–194
    and periodontal disease, 199, 201
    preventing, 85, 87, 95, 114–115
    stress leading to, 174–175
    for weight fluctuations, 28
Heliotropium and barbiturates, 70
Herbal remedies, 69–71, 91–93, 97, 99,
    100
Heritage, x–xi
Hernandez, Manuel "Manny," 177–179
High blood pressure (hypertension)
    chubby childhood leading to, 21
    and dietary supplements, 70, 79, 86, 91
    and exercise, 106, 137, 141–142, 153
    medications for, 168, 197, 198
    statistics on diabetes and, 194
    and waist-to-hip ratio, 25
    and walking the dog, 180
High blood sugar. *See* Hyperglycemia
High-fiber, unrefined diet, 65–66
High-GI carbohydrates, 53, 125–126, 185
Hispanics, xiii–xiv. *See also* Latinos
Hispanopolis, 19
Honey for diabetic foot ulcers, 98–99

Hormones
  amylin, 155, 160, 162–163
  endorphins, 180
  from fat cells, 24
  glucose-raising, from exercise, 102–104
  incretin hormones, 157–158
Humalog, 164–165
Humulin N, 164–165, 167
Humulin R, 164, 165
Hydration tips for exercise, 130
Hydrogenated oils, 48
Hyperglycemia
  and B vitamins, 78
  and exercise, 104–105, 120
  and gastroparesis, 197
  and medications, 156, 158–159, 164
  and nutritional supplements, 72, 83–84
  symptoms of, 2
Hyperinsulinemia, 23
Hypertension. *See* High blood pressure
Hypoglycemia
  causes and symptoms, 123–125
  and exercise, 120, 162–163, 167
  and gastroparesis, 139, 197
  and medications, 156, 157, 160, 161,
    162–163
  preventing, 128
  traveling and, 204
  treatments, 125–127
Hypoglycemia unawareness, 127–128
Hyponatremia, 130–131

Immune system, 3–4, 74, 174
Impaired fasting glucose (IFG), 4, 6, 8
Impaired glucose tolerance (IGT), 6, 8
Impaired sensation, 195. *See also* Peripheral
  neuropathy
Incretin hormones, 157–158
Incretins and incretin mimetics, 155,
  160–161
Inflammation in joints or tendons, 97
Inflammatory diet, 41, 48, 50
Inflammatory process, 48, 175, 218
Injuries during exercise, treatment for,
  144–145
Insoluble fiber, 47

Insulin
  and carbohydrates, 40–41, 53
  effect of exercise, 104–106, 113–115,
    123
  and exercise, 166
  ketones from lack of, 129
  for lowering blood sugar at rest, 104
  overview, 163–166
  syringes for, 166, 177–178, 202, 203, 204
  traveling with, 202–204
Insulin action, 8, 35, 104, 164–165, 167
Insulin and insulin analogs action, 165
Insulin autoantibodies, 4
Insulin pumpers club, 178
Insulin resistance
  and blood glucose uptake, 26
  from caffeine, 64
  controlling nutrient deficiencies from, 72
  and depressive symptoms, 175
  from excess free radicals, 73
  exercise versus, 104–105
  foods leading to, 48–49
  high-GI values leading to, 54
  by the liver, 27
  overview, 7–8
  smoking and, 218
  in type 2 diabetes and prediabetes, 2, 3,
    34–36
Insulin sensitivity, 47, 64, 66, 96, 114
Insulin-to-carbohydrate ratio, 56
Insulite Laboratories diabetes management
    system, 17
Integrated Diabetes Services, 17
Inter-esterified fat, 52
Intermediate-action insulin, 164–165,
  167
International travel, 202–204
Internet resources, 17–19, 42–43, 50,
  53–54, 94, 223–226
Interval training, 115–116
Iron, 88
Ischemia, 134–135, 139

Joint-related injuries or pain, 97, 117,
  143–144
Jonas, Nick, 215

Joslin Diabetes Center (Boston), 42–43
Journals, 217

Ketosis, 129
Kidneys, 87, 95, 142–143, 194–195, 197
Knowledge about diabetes management, 133, 178, 187, 200, 208

Labels on packaged foods, reading, 47, 61, 107–108
Lactilol, 62
LADA (latent autoimmune diabetes of the adult), 3–4, 165
Lantus, 164, 165, 167
Lard, cooking with, x
Latinos
    barriers to exercising, 102, 200
    barriers to managing diabetes, 14–15, 60, 149, 196
    challenges of educating, 207–208
    diet and diabetes control, 37–40, 65–66
    English language barrier, 13–14
    ethnic group classification, xiii–xiv
    failure to recognize and treat depression, 175–176
    HbA1c values, 14, 149, 196
    knowledge about diabetes, 133, 178, 187, 200
    Latino-style foods with low GI, 47, 52–53, 56, 59–60
    statistics on diabetes, ix, xiv–xv, 195–196, 201
    See also Cultural heritage; Family
Laughter, benefits from, 173
L-carnitine, 96–97
LDL cholesterol, 48–49, 51, 90
Leg pain, exercising with, 136–137
Legumes, 44, 56
Lemonade, sugar-sweetened, 61
Leptin, 24
Leucine, 96
Levemir, 164, 165, 167
Lidocaine, 98
Lifestyle choices
    eating breakfast, 66
    effect of healthy modifications, 196

Latina's secrets for, 133
living with diabetes and helping others, 84–85, 107–108, 131–133, 177–179, 187–188, 200, 214–215
maintaining healthy changes, 119, 211, 212–214
overview, 8–9, 22–23, 30–31
without sugar, 60–63
See also Cultural heritage; Diabetes management
Linoleic acid, conjugated, 72
Lipid levels test, 72–73, 122, 137
Lipitor, 82, 153, 167–168
Lipoic acid (LA), 73–74, 82–83, 98
Liver, 26–27, 51, 103
Low blood pressure, 168
Low blood sugar. *See* Hypoglycemia
Low-fat diets, 31, 39, 51, 63
Lutein, 43–44
Lycopene, 43–44
Lyrica, 197

Macular degeneration, 83
Magnesium, 74, 86–87, 88
Mannitol, 62
Martinez de Pozos, Maria de los Angeles, 159
Meats, 48, 49
Medical treatments, 99–100, 197–199, 201–202
Medications
    administration of, 166–167
    amylin, 155, 160, 162–163
    changing from oral to insulin, 177–178
    combination therapies, 154, 156, 158–160, 164–165
    Coumadin, 82, 92, 169, 199
    and exercise, 125, 161–162, 167–168
    Lipitor, 82, 153, 167–168
    metformin, 11, 153–154, 155, 156–157
    overview, 153–156
    pramlintide, 155, 160, 162–163
    Reglan, 197
    self-prescribing supplements warning, 70–71

Medications (*continued*)
  side effects, 133, 142, 156–157, 167–168, 197–198
  taking as prescribed, 133
  tPA, 199
  See also Aspirin therapy; Doctors
Medications, types of
  ACE-inhibitors, 168, 197
  alpha-glucosidase inhibitors, 155, 158, 162
  angiotensin receptor blockers, 197
  anticoagulants, 199
  anti-inflammatory, 97, 144, 145, 199
  antiplatelet agents, 198, 199
  beta-blockers, 168
  biguanides, 11, 153–154, 155, 156–157
  blood thinners, 82, 91, 92, 169
  diuretics, 168
  DPP-4 inhibitors, 155, 157–158
  incretins and incretin mimetics, 155, 160–161
  meglitinides/phenylalanine derivatives, 155, 158, 162
  for nerve pain, 197
  statins, 153, 167–168
  sulfonylureas, 154, 155, 156, 161–162
  thiazolidinediones, 154, 155, 157, 162
  vasodilators, 168
  See also Insulin
Meglitinides/phenylalanine derivatives, 155, 158, 162
Memory and gingko biloba, 91–92
Mental control, 159
Mental outlook. *See* Positive mental outlook
Mental stress, 10, 175–176. *See also* Emotions; Stress
Metabolic acidosis, 129
Metabolic syndrome, 117
Metabolism
  and B vitamins, 75, 78, 183
  effect of diabetes, 72
  kick-starting with breakfast, 66
  L-carnitine for fats and carbohydrates, 96–97
  and magnesium, 86
  and zinc, 89–90
Metformin, 11, 153–154, 155, 156–157
Mevacor, 153, 167–168
Mexican Americans, ix, xiv–xv, 102. *See also* Latinos
Mexico, 85
Mexico Diabetes Federation, 84
Microalbumin excretions and exercise, 142–143
Micronase, 154, 155, 156, 161–162
Milk for hypoglycemia treatment, 127
Moderation versus supersizing, 185
Monitoring your blood sugar
  exercising and, 123–124, 141
  as GPS of diabetes, 59–60
  importance of, 84, 107–108, 132, 150–151
  overview, 11
  and supplement intake, 72–73
  See also Blood glucose levels
Monounsaturated fats, 51
Mugwort and dermatitis, 70
Muscle mass, losing, 114–115, 217
Muscles
  exercise and glycogen in, 7–8, 34–35, 58, 103–104, 217
  fat storage in, 26
  glucose storage in, 35–36
  insulin action in, 35, 104
  slow-twitch and fast-twitch fibers, 113–114
  soreness due to exercise, 144–146
  stress proteins in, 144
Myths and beliefs in Latino culture, 15–16, 208

N (intermediate-action insulin), 164–165, 167
National Academy of Sciences, 81
National Institutes of Health, 94
National Weight Control Registry, 28–29
Natural killer (NK) cells, 74
Nephropathy, 87, 95, 142–143, 194–195, 197

Nerve damage, 139–140, 195. *See also*
  Peripheral neuropathy
Nerve fiber regeneration, 83
Neurontin, 197
Neuropathy. *See* Peripheral neuropathy
Niacin, 75, 76, 78
Nitroglycerin, 168
NK (natural killer) cells, 74
Norepinephrine, 103
NovoLog, 164–165
NutraSweet (aspartame), 62
Nutrient density of foods, 94
Nutrition labels, reading, 47, 61, 107–108

Obesity, 7–8, 14, 21, 23–26, 36. *See also*
  Overweight adults
OGTT (oral glucose tolerance test), 6, 7
Oils, 49, 51–52
Olive oil, 49, 51
Omega-3 essential fats, 49, 52, 183
Omega-6 essential fats, 49–50
Ophthalmologists, 142, 198
Optimists and pessimists, 40-year study of,
  172
Oral glucose tolerance test (OGTT), 6, 7
Oral hygiene, 199, 201
Orange-yellow foods, 44, 74–75
Organically-grown products, 49, 50
Orinase, 154, 155, 156, 161–162
Orthostatic hypotension, 139, 195
Overhydration, 130–131
Overweight adults
  effect of low-GI diet on, 54–55
  emotional concerns from, 175
  fitness as priority, 23–24, 28, 29, 101,
    118
  obesity, 7–8, 14, 21, 23–26, 36
  overcoming barrier to exercise, 110–112
  and risk of arthritis, 143–144
  from sedentary lifestyle, 33–34, 106
Overweight children, 21, 23, 27
Oxidative stress, 41, 44–45, 73

PAD (peripheral artery disease), 136–137
Pancreatic beta cells, 2, 3, 90, 165, 179
Pantothenic acid, 75, 77, 78

Pedometers, 146, 208–209
Pens for insulin, 166
Periodontal disease, 199, 201
Peripheral artery disease (PAD), 136–137
Peripheral neuropathy
  alpha lipoic acid for treating, 83
  autonomic nerve damage, 139–140, 195
  exercising safely with, 138–139
  medical treatments for, 197–198
  pain relief, 78, 92–93, 98, 99
  smoking and, 218
  treatments for, 97, 98
  vitamin C for preventing, 79
Pessimists and optimists, 40-year study of,
  172
Pets and emotional fitness, 180–181
Phosphorus, 89
Physical activity, 179–180, 208–209. *See
  also* Exercise
Phytochemicals (phytonutrients), 43–45,
  97
Pick up the pace (PUP) training, 115–116
Pima Native Americans, 22–23
Plavix, 199
Polysaccharides (fiber), 46–48, 65–66
Popcorn, 55
Portion size, calories, and carbohydrates
  list, 57–58
Positive mental outlook
  effect of food on mood, 182–183
  emotional fitness through physical
    activity, 179–180
  involving family in your diabetes care,
    186–189
  managing stress and, 171–174
  moderation versus supersizing, 185
  overview, 171, 189
  pets and, 180–181
  and physical well-being, 176, 181–182,
    218
  reducing stress, 172
  See also Exercise; Healthy eating;
    Lifestyle choices
Potassium, 88
Pramlintide, 155, 160, 162–163
Prandin, 155, 158, 162

Pravachol, 153, 167–168
Precose, 155, 158, 162
Prediabetes, 6, 7–8, 117–118. *See also*
    Insulin resistance
Pregnancy with diabetes, 85, 158,
    201–202
Processed foods
    avoiding bingeing on, 183
    at fast food restaurants, 34, 41, 48–49
    fat-free and sugar-free foods, 61–62
    fiber refined out of, 47
    glycemic effect, 43
    high-GI values of, 53, 60
    saturated and trans fats in, 48
    unhealthy fats in, 51
Procyanidines, 91
Produce, availability of native, xi
Proliferative diabetic retinopathy, xvi, 75,
    140–142, 194, 198
Propionyl-L-carnitine, 96–97
Protein excretions and exercise, 142–143
Protein intake, 94–95, 197
Puberty, 4
Puerto Ricans, xiv–xv. *See also* Latinos
Pumps for insulin, 166–167
Punishment for personal sins, 15–16
PUP (pick up the pace) training, 115–116
Purple-blue foods, 44
Pycnogenol, 91
Pyridoxine (B6), 75, 77, 78

Quercetin, 43–44, 97

Range of motion, 97, 116
Rapid-acting insulin analog, 164–165
Red foods, 44
Reglan, 197
Regular (Humulin R), 164, 165
Relapse recovery, 60
Religion, 12–13
Resistance exercise, 95–96, 212
Resistance to change, overcoming,
    216–217
Resources in print, 18, 231–232. *See also*
    Internet resources
Reverse weight gain, 28–30, 31

Rewarding yourself for success, 215–216
Riboflavin (B2), 75, 76, 78
RICE techniques (rest, ice, compression,
    and elevation), 145
Riomet, 155, 156–157
Rodriguez, Gloria, 9–12
Rojas, Thaylu, 214–215
Rojas de Chacin, Gladys, 200

Saponins, 43–44
Saturated fats, 48, 51, 52
Sedentary lifestyles, 33–34, 210
Selenium, 73–74, 87, 88
Self-care on bad days, 216–217
Self-prescribing supplements, 70–71
Shooting pains, 195
Side effects of medications, 133, 142,
    156–157, 167–168, 197
Smoking and gum disease, 201
Smoking cessation, 137, 181, 218–219
Sodium, 89
Soft drinks, 61
Soluble fiber, 47
Sorbitol, 62
Soups, broth-based, 65
Soy protein, 94–95
Spikes in blood glucose
    from carbohydrates, 35–36, 41, 56, 183
    controlling/preventing, 41–42, 120, 150,
        158
    and estimated average glucose, 152
    and glycemic index, 53–55
    laughter and, 173
    from low-fiber foods, 48
Splenda (sucralose), 62
Sports drinks, 130, 131
Starlix, 155, 158, 162
Statins, 153, 167–168
Statistics
    on activity-related injuries, 111
    on caffeine-induced glucose spikes, 64
    on diabetes and hypertension, 194
    on diabetes in Latino Americans, ix,
        xiv–xv, 195–196, 201
    exercise in America, 33
    on need for insulin, 163

obesity in the United States, 23
uninsured Latinos in the United States, 14
Stress, 132–133, 172–173, 174–175
Stress proteins, 144
Stretching, 110, 116–117, 143–144
Stroke, 193, 199, 201
Sucralose (Splenda), 62
Sugar, 60–63, 182–183
Sugar alcohols, 62
Sugar equivalents on nutrition labels, 61
Sugar-free foods, 61–62
Sulfonylureas, 154, 155, 156, 161–162
Sulforaphane, 44
Sunlight, vitamin D from exposure to, 80–81
Supplements
  finding nutrient content in, 94
  need for, 71–73
  overdosing dangers, 74, 75, 78, 99
  overview, 69, 100
  self-prescribing, warning about, 70, 71
  See also specific vitamins and minerals
Sweeteners, artificial or low-calorie, 62
Swimming or pool exercises, 111–112, 138
Symlin, 155, 160, 162–163
Symptoms
  of depression, 175, 179
  of diabetes, 2–4, 5, 84, 107, 117
  of gastroparesis, 195, 197
  of heart attack, 135, 136
  of hyperglycemia, 2
  of hypoglycemia, 124, 127
  of ischemia, 134–135, 139
  of nerve damage, 195, 198–199
  of neuropathy, 97–98
  of orthostatic hypertension, 195
  of PAD, 136
  of prediabetes, 117
  of stroke, 199
Syringes, 166, 177–178, 202, 203, 204

Taking Control of Your Diabetes Latino Initiative, 17, 19
Tea, 45, 61
Television shows targeting Latinos, 11

Television watching, negative effects of, 33–34
Tendonitis, 97, 117, 143–144
Terpenes, 43–44
Thiamin (B1), 75, 76, 78
Thiazolidinediones (TZDs), 154, 155, 157, 162
Thoughts, changing your, 173. *See also* Positive mental outlook
Tibetan Buddhist monks, 174
Time constraints to caring for yourself, 84
Tips
  dietary sources of essential vitamins and minerals, 76–77, 88–89
  for exercising safely, 109, 116, 122, 130, 141, 146
  finding nutrient content of foods and supplements, 94
  heart attack warning signs, 136
  keeping lifestyle change motivation strong, 211
  for maintaining mental function, 182
  portion size, calories, and carb content of common foods, 57–58
  preparing healthier meals, 45–46
  preventing hypoglycemia, 128
  relaxing and reducing stress, 172
  sources of carbohydrates for hypoglycemia, 126
  strategies for controlling blood sugar, 63
  target goals for tests, 154
  for traveling with diabetes, 203
  on workout DVDs, 112–113
Tocopherol compounds, 81–82
Toothbrush trauma, 201
Topical creams for painful neuropathy, 98
TPA (clot-busting drug), 199
Trans fats, 48, 51, 52
Transportation Security Administration (TSA), 203
Traveling with diabetes, 202–204
Trigger fingers, 97, 117, 143–144
Trigger point massage, 97
Triglycerides, 48
TuDiabetes.com community, 178

Type 1 diabetes
  characteristics of people with, 5
  and insulin, 163, 165
  and insulin autoantibodies, 4
  living with and helping others, 84–85,
    107–108, 177–179, 214–215
  overview, 2, 3–4
  vitamin D deficiency as contributor, 80
Type 1.5 diabetes (LADA), 3–4, 165
Type 2 diabetes
  characteristics of people with, 5
  effect of low-GI diet, 55
  and elevated fasting insulin, 4
  and exercise, 106, 114, 122
  incidence of need for insulin, 163
  living with and helping others, 131–133,
    187–188, 200
  obesity and, 23
  overview, 2–3, 19
  preventability of, xv
  and soy protein, 95
  and vitamin C deficiency, 79

United States, ix, xiii, xiv–xv, 23
U.S. Transportation Security
  Administration (TSA), 203

Vanadium and vanadyl sulfate, 87, 89
Vasodilators, 168
Vegetables, 43–45, 53, 65, 83, 212
Venezuela, 200, 214–215
Visceral fat, 21–22, 24–26, 118. *See also*
  Body fat
Vitamin A (retinol), 74, 75, 76
Vitamin B2 (riboflavin), 75, 76, 78
Vitamin B6 (pyridoxine), 75, 77, 78
Vitamin B12, 77
Vitamin C (ascorbic acid), 73–74, 77, 79

Vitamin D (calcitriol), 76, 80–81, 98
Vitamin E, 73–74, 76, 81–82
Vitamin K, 77
Vitamins, dietary sources of, 76–77. *See
  also* Supplements; *specific vitamins*

Waist-to-hip ratio (WHR), 25–26
Walking
  with arthritis, 143–144
  bad weather back-up plan, 209
  with diabetes complications, 135, 137
  for diabetes prevention, 30–32
  dog walking vs. gym workouts,
    180–181
  muscular activity during, 104–105
  self-confidence from, 111
  sitting versus, 106
Water intake, 129–131
Water intoxication, 130–131
Watermelon, 55
Weight gain as early symptom of diabetes,
  117
Weight loss
  effect of, 27
  with exercise, 24, 30–31, 117–119
  fitness as priority over, 23–24, 28, 29,
    101, 118
  keeping the weight off, 28–30, 31
  with low GI/GL diet plan, 56
  See also Exercise; Healthy eating
Weight training, 103, 113–115, 135,
  141–142
White foods, 44
White vinegar, 94
Workout DVDs, 112–113

Zinc, 73–74, 88, 89–90
Zocor, 153, 167–168